DASH DIET COOKBOOK FOR BEGINNERS

1800 Days of Simple, Scrumptious Recipes that Reduce Blood Pressure and Stimulate Weight Loss. Includes a 60-Day Food Plan

Alysia Jordan

Table of Contents

CHAPTER 1: INTRODUCTION TO THE DASH DIET
1.1 THE ORIGINS AND SCIENCE BEHIND THE DASH DIET

The journey to discovering the DASH (Dietary Approaches to Stop Hypertension) diet is like uncovering a hidden gem in the vast landscape of nutritional science. Its origins date back to the early 1990s, when researchers observed the profound impact of dietary patterns on blood pressure and overall cardiovascular health. The DASH diet emerged from a series of studies funded by the National Institutes of Health (NIH) that sought to identify the dietary elements playing pivotal roles in blood pressure regulation.

Imagine scientists, much like culinary detectives, meticulously analyzing the effects of various foods and nutrients on heart health. Their investigation led to a groundbreaking discovery: a diet rich in fruits, vegetables, whole grains, and lean proteins could significantly lower blood pressure, thereby reducing the risk of heart disease, stroke, and kidney problems.

The original DASH study was more than just a clinical trial; it was a beacon of hope for millions grappling with hypertension. Participants who followed the DASH diet experienced a remarkable reduction in blood pressure, sometimes even within just two weeks, comparable to the effects of medication. The diet's high intake of potassium, magnesium, calcium, and fiber, alongside low sodium levels, was credited for these impressive results.

Delving deeper into the science, the DASH diet's efficacy is rooted in its nutrient-rich components that work synergistically to improve heart health. Potassium, for example, helps balance the amount of sodium in cells, essential for maintaining healthy blood pressure levels. Magnesium and calcium play crucial roles in cardiovascular function, aiding in the regulation of blood flow and nerve signal transmission.

Beyond its immediate impact on blood pressure, the DASH diet has shown promise in addressing other health concerns, such as aiding weight loss, improving insulin sensitivity, and reducing the risk of certain cancers and diabetes. Its comprehensive nature makes it more than a diet—it's a sustainable approach to eating that nurtures the body holistically.

The adaptability of the DASH diet is one of its most compelling features. It's not a rigid plan but a flexible eating pattern that can be tailored to individual tastes, lifestyles, and nutritional needs. This versatility makes it accessible and sustainable for a wide range of people, from busy parents and professionals to seniors and athletes. The diet encourages whole, nutrient-dense foods while allowing for variety and flavor, making it easier to stick to in the long run.

What sets the DASH diet apart in the world of nutrition is its evidence-based foundation and its holistic approach to health. It's not just about lowering blood pressure; it's about setting the stage for a healthier lifestyle that can lead to lasting change. The diet's principles encourage mindful eating and a deeper understanding of how food affects our bodies, promoting a harmonious relationship between diet and health.

Integrating the DASH diet into daily life doesn't require drastic changes. It starts with small, manageable adjustments, like incorporating more fruits and vegetables into meals, choosing whole grains, and selecting lean protein sources. Over time, these changes can become a natural part of one's eating habits, leading to improved health and well-being.

The success stories of individuals who have adopted the DASH diet are both inspiring and affirming. From significant blood pressure improvements to weight loss and enhanced energy levels, these personal tales underscore the diet's potential to transform lives. They serve as a testament to the power of dietary choices in influencing health and provide a source of motivation for others embarking on their own health journeys.

The DASH diet's ongoing evolution reflects the dynamic nature of nutritional science. As new research emerges, the diet continues to be refined and updated, ensuring it remains relevant and effective in promoting heart health and overall well-being. This adaptability and commitment to evidence-based practice have solidified the DASH diet's reputation as one of the most effective and sustainable dietary approaches for preventing and managing hypertension and fostering long-term health.

In essence, the DASH diet transcends the conventional concept of dieting. It represents a holistic paradigm shift in how we view food and its impact on our health. By emphasizing nutrient-dense foods and balanced eating patterns, the DASH diet offers a practical, enjoyable, and scientifically backed path to improved health and vitality. Its origins and evolution in the realm of nutritional science not only highlight the critical role of diet in managing hypertension but also underscore the broader potential of informed dietary choices to enhance our overall quality of life.

1.2 KEY BENEFITS OF THE DASH DIET

Embarking on the DASH (Dietary Approaches to Stop Hypertension) diet journey unveils a spectrum of benefits that transcend mere blood pressure reduction. It's akin to discovering a treasure chest of health gems, each with its unique sparkle contributing to a more vibrant, healthier you.

At its core, the DASH diet is lauded for its significant impact on blood pressure levels. Imagine the relief and empowerment of seeing those numbers drop without the sole reliance on medication. This is the reality for many who follow the DASH diet, as it naturally encourages the reduction of sodium intake while increasing nutrients like potassium, calcium, and magnesium—key players in the cardiovascular symphony that helps manage blood pressure.

But the magic of the DASH diet doesn't stop there. Its holistic approach to nutrition has far-reaching benefits beyond the heart's arteries. For instance, weight management becomes more attainable with this diet. It promotes foods that are rich in fiber and low in unhealthy fats and sugars, which can naturally lead to a calorie deficit without the need for strict calorie counting or portion control. It's about feeling full and satisfied, not deprived, making sustainable weight loss a more accessible goal.

Moreover, the diet's emphasis on whole foods and diverse nutrients has a ripple effect on various aspects of health, including metabolic syndrome, diabetes, and inflammation. By adopting a DASH-friendly eating pattern, individuals often experience improved insulin sensitivity and a decrease in insulin resistance, cornerstones in preventing and managing type 2 diabetes. The diet's rich array of antioxidants and anti-inflammatory foods also plays a crucial role in combating oxidative stress and inflammation, underlying factors in many chronic diseases.

Heart health, while a primary focus, is just one of the many areas where the DASH diet shines. Its nutrient-dense framework supports a robust cardiovascular system, reducing the risk of heart disease, stroke, and even some forms of cancer. This is because the diet's foundation—fruits, vegetables, whole grains, and lean proteins—provides a plethora of essential nutrients that fortify the body's defenses against these conditions.

But what makes the DASH diet genuinely remarkable is its adaptability and how it fits into the tapestry of daily life. It's not just a diet but a lifestyle choice that emphasizes balanced, enjoyable eating. There's no need for exotic ingredients or complicated recipes; the DASH diet is grounded in simplicity and accessibility, making it feasible for anyone, regardless of culinary skill or budget. Mental health and cognitive function also reap the benefits of the DASH diet. Nutrient-rich foods, particularly those high in omega-3 fatty acids, antioxidants, and phytonutrients, have been linked to improved mood and cognitive performance. Following this dietary pattern can contribute to better mental clarity, reduced risk of depression, and a potential slowdown in cognitive decline as we age.

The inclusive nature of the DASH diet means it can be customized to fit various cultural preferences and dictary restrictions, making it a universally appealing choice. Whether you are a vegetarian, have food allergies, or prefer certain cuisines, the DASH diet can be tailored to meet your needs while still adhering to its core principles of health and nutrition.

In essence, the DASH diet is not just about reducing sodium or preventing hypertension. It's about nurturing the body, mind, and spirit with nutritious, whole foods that offer a cascade of health benefits. This diet champions the idea that what we eat significantly impacts our overall health and well-being, advocating for a balanced, mindful approach to eating.

Through its versatile and holistic nature, the DASH diet empowers individuals to take control of their health and embark on a journey to a more fulfilled, healthier life. It's a testament to the power of dietary choices in shaping our health destiny, offering a path to wellness that is both nourishing and sustainable. In embracing the DASH diet, we embrace a lifestyle that prioritizes health without sacrificing pleasure, ensuring that each meal is a step towards a healthier future.

1.3 HOW TO START YOUR DASH DIET JOURNEY

Beginning your DASH diet journey is like embarking on a new adventure, one that leads to better health and well-being. It's a path that requires guidance, commitment, and a dash of enthusiasm to explore new foods and flavors. Let's delve into how you can start this transformative journey, step by step, with practicality and pleasure intertwined.

The first step is understanding that the DASH diet is more than just a list of foods to eat and avoid; it's a lifestyle change aimed at promoting heart health and overall well-being. This means adopting a holistic approach to eating that includes a variety of nutrient-rich foods, while also considering portion sizes and meal timing.

To ease into the DASH diet, start by gradually increasing your intake of fruits and vegetables. These should be the stars of your meals, filling your plate with a rainbow of colors and a wealth of vitamins, minerals, and fibers. Think of it as adding more nature to your diet, where each color represents a different nutrient or health benefit, making your meals not only visually appealing but also nutritionally comprehensive.

Whole grains are another cornerstone of the DASH diet. Replacing refined grains like white bread and pasta with whole-grain alternatives such as brown rice, quinoa, and whole-wheat pasta introduces more fiber to your diet, which aids digestion and helps you feel full longer. It's a simple switch with substantial benefits for your heart and waistline.

Lean proteins, including fish, poultry, beans, and nuts, are essential for building and repairing tissues and should be included in your diet in moderation. These protein sources provide the necessary building blocks for your body, without the excess fat and calories often found in red meats and processed foods.

Dairy is also part of the DASH diet, but it's advisable to opt for low-fat or fat-free versions to get the calcium and vitamin D you need without the extra saturated fat. This helps maintain bone strength while supporting heart health.

One of the most critical aspects of the DASH diet is managing sodium intake. High sodium consumption is a key player in hypertension, so reducing salt in your diet is paramount. Start by cooking more at home, where you can control the amount of salt added to your food. Use herbs and spices to flavor your dishes instead of salt, and be mindful of sodium content in processed foods by reading labels carefully.

Hydration is another vital element of the DASH diet. Drinking plenty of water helps maintain optimal bodily functions and can also aid in reducing sodium levels through urination. Incorporate water-rich foods like cucumbers, tomatoes, and watermelon into your diet to help stay hydrated.

Beginning the DASH diet also means paying attention to your eating habits. Eating slowly and mindfully allows you to enjoy your food more and gives your body time to signal when it's full, preventing overeating. Planning meals and snacks ahead of time can also help you stay on track, making it easier to avoid unhealthy food choices.

As you start your DASH diet journey, remember that gradual changes are more sustainable than drastic ones. You don't have to overhaul your diet overnight. Small, consistent modifications to your eating habits can lead to significant health benefits over time. For example, adding one serving of vegetables to your dinner each night or switching to whole-grain bread for your morning toast can set the foundation for more substantial changes.

The beauty of the DASH diet lies in its flexibility and adaptability. It's not about strict rules or deprivation but about finding a balanced and enjoyable way of eating that can be maintained for life. This approach ensures that the diet is not only effective in the short term but also sustainable in the long term, leading to lasting health benefits.

Engaging with a supportive community, whether online or in person, can also enhance your DASH diet journey. Sharing experiences, recipes, and tips with others who are on the same path can provide motivation and inspiration, making the journey more enjoyable and successful.

Finally, consulting with healthcare professionals like a dietitian can provide personalized guidance to ensure that the DASH diet meets your specific health needs and goals. They can help tailor the diet to your preferences, making it easier to stick to and more effective in achieving your health objectives.

In conclusion, starting your DASH diet journey is about embracing a healthier lifestyle through mindful, balanced eating and gradual, sustainable changes. By focusing on nutrient-rich foods, managing sodium intake, and enjoying the variety and flavors of a heart-healthy diet, you can embark on a path to improved health and well-being. It's a journey that requires commitment and adaptation, but with the right approach and support, it's a journey that can be both rewarding and delicious.

CHAPTER 2: UNDERSTANDING NUTRIENTS & PLANNING YOUR MEALS

2.1 A CLOSER LOOK AT SODIUM, POTASSIUM, AND OTHER ESSENTIAL NUTRIENTS

Delving into the world of essential nutrients, especially in the context of the DASH diet, is like embarking on a fascinating journey through the building blocks of our body's health. Sodium, potassium, and other vital nutrients play leading roles in this narrative, each with its unique contributions to our well-being.

Sodium often takes center stage in discussions about diet and health, particularly regarding blood pressure and heart health. It's a mineral that's crucial for maintaining fluid balance in the body, aiding in nerve function, and influencing muscle contractions. However, the modern diet tends to tip the scales with excessive sodium intake, leading to hypertension and cardiovascular risks. The DASH diet's approach to sodium is not about complete elimination but finding a healthier balance. It encourages reducing processed and high-salt foods while savoring the natural flavors of whole, unprocessed ingredients, thereby naturally lowering sodium intake without sacrificing taste.

On the other side of the spectrum is potassium, a mineral that plays a complementary role to sodium. Potassium helps relax blood vessel walls, thus lowering blood pressure and countering some of sodium's adverse effects. It's abundant in fruits, vegetables, and legumes, making these foods staples in the DASH diet. The beauty of focusing on these potassium-rich foods is that they offer more than just this single nutrient; they bring a symphony of vitamins, minerals, and antioxidants, all contributing to overall health and preventing various chronic conditions.

But the nutrient story doesn't end with just sodium and potassium. Calcium is another star in the DASH diet's nutrient ensemble, known primarily for its role in bone health. Yet, its influence extends to cardiovascular health as well, helping to regulate blood pressure alongside its partners. Low-fat dairy products, fortified plant-based alternatives, leafy greens, and almonds are excellent calcium sources, aligning perfectly with the DASH diet's guidelines.

Magnesium, though less talked about, is no less important. This nutrient aids in hundreds of biochemical reactions in the body, including those that regulate blood pressure. Magnesium-rich foods like whole grains, nuts, seeds, and legumes are prominent in the DASH diet, seamlessly integrating this vital mineral into daily meals.

Exploring these nutrients reveals the intricacies of how our bodies function and the profound impact our dietary choices have on our health. The DASH diet, with its emphasis on these essential nutrients, showcases a holistic approach to eating. It's not just about reducing sodium or increasing potassium; it's about creating a balanced and nutritious dietary pattern that supports overall health.

Understanding these nutrients' roles and sources enables us to make informed choices about our meals. It's not about stringent rules or strict diets but about knowledge and balance. For example, instead of simply cutting out salty snacks, we can replace them with nuts or seeds, which are high in potassium and magnesium, offering a double benefit for blood pressure management.

The narrative of nutrients in the DASH diet is one of harmony and balance, where each element plays a part in the larger story of health and well-being. It's a story that weaves together the scientific and the practical, showing us that our everyday food choices can have a significant impact on our health. This understanding empowers us to make decisions that support our body's needs, aligning with the DASH diet's principles to foster a healthier, more vibrant life.

In this journey through the world of essential nutrients, we learn that each meal is an opportunity to nourish our bodies, improve our health, and enjoy the pleasures of delicious, wholesome foods. The DASH diet, with its focus on these key nutrients, offers a guide to making those opportunities count, leading us towards a healthier heart and a fuller life.

2.2 READING FOOD LABELS AND MAKING HEALTHIER CHOICES

Navigating the world of food labels can feel like deciphering a complex map, but understanding this language is key to making healthier choices that align with the DASH diet. Let's embark on a journey through the maze of nutritional information, learning to read food labels not as a tedious chore but as a powerful tool to guide our dietary decisions. When you pick up a packaged food item, the nutrition facts label is your window into its nutritional value, offering insights into its components like sodium, fats, sugars, and other essential nutrients. To make healthier choices, the first stop on this label-reading journey is the sodium content. The DASH diet emphasizes low sodium intake to manage blood pressure, so identifying foods with lower sodium levels is crucial. Look for labels that show lower percentages of daily value (%DV) for sodium, ideally less than 5%. Next, your gaze might fall on the fats section. But not all fats are foes; it's the type of fat that matters. The DASH diet favors heart-healthy fats, such as monounsaturated and polyunsaturated fats, over saturated and trans fats. Foods with higher levels of unsaturated fats and lower levels of saturated and trans fats are more in line with DASH principles, supporting heart health and overall well-being. Carbohydrates, often vilified in diet culture, are actually an essential energy source. The key is choosing the right type of carbs. Whole grains, a staple of the DASH diet, are rich in fiber and nutrients, offering a steadier source of energy and helping maintain blood sugar levels. When reading labels, look for higher fiber content and whole grain ingredients listed at the beginning of the ingredient list, indicating a healthier, more DASH-friendly choice. Sugar, particularly added sugar, is another critical point on food labels. The DASH diet encourages reducing added sugars, which can be hidden in many products. Labels now differentiate between total sugars and added sugars, allowing you to see how much sugar is naturally occurring and how much has been added. Opting for foods with low or no added sugars can significantly impact your health, reducing risks of diabetes, obesity, and heart disease. Protein is an essential component of the DASH diet, providing the building blocks for muscles and tissues. The label can help you choose lean protein sources, such as poultry, fish, beans, and nuts, which are integral to the DASH eating plan. Checking the protein content can guide you in selecting foods that contribute to your daily protein needs without excessive saturated fat. Beyond these specific nutrients, the ingredient list on a food label offers a wealth of information about the food's quality and nutritional value. Ingredients are listed in order of quantity, from highest to lowest. A DASH-friendly product will have whole foods, like fruits, vegetables, whole grains, and lean proteins, listed at the beginning, indicating that they are the main ingredients. Understanding serving sizes and servings per container is also vital in making healthier choices. What might seem like a DASH-compatible food could become less so if the serving size is small and you consume multiple servings. This awareness can help you manage portion sizes, a key aspect of the DASH diet and overall healthy eating. In the journey of making healthier food choices, knowledge is power. Reading food labels empowers you to discern what's truly in your food, enabling you to select products that align with the DASH diet and your health goals. This practice becomes less of a task and more of an informed decision-making process, where you choose foods based on a deep understanding of their nutritional content and impact on your health. The narrative of reading food labels is like uncovering the story behind each product, revealing the truth beyond marketing claims and packaging allure. It's about becoming a savvy consumer who can navigate the supermarket aisles with confidence, armed with the knowledge to make choices that contribute to a healthier, happier life. In this context, the DASH diet becomes more than a set of guidelines; it's a framework for making informed, mindful food choices that support your journey to better health. Reading food labels with a discerning eye is a skill that enhances this journey, allowing you to take control of your dietary habits and embrace a lifestyle that fosters well-being and vitality.

2.3 CREATING A BALANCED DASH PLATE PORTION SIZES AND FOOD GROUPINGS

Creating a balanced DASH plate is akin to painting a masterpiece, where each element plays a critical role in the overall composition. It's about more than just the individual colors—or in this case, food groups—it's how they blend together to create a harmonious and nourishing meal. The DASH diet emphasizes variety and balance, guiding us to fill our plates with a rich tapestry of colors, textures, and nutrients. To achieve this, envision your plate divided into sections, each representing different food groups that together form a balanced meal. Half of your plate should be a vibrant array of fruits and vegetables, the cornerstone of the DASH diet. These nutrient-dense foods are high in fiber, vitamins, and minerals, and low in calories, making them ideal for managing blood pressure and supporting overall health. Imagine leafy greens, bright bell peppers, juicy berries, and crisp apples, creating a colorful and appetizing display. This abundance of fruits and vegetables not only nourishes the body but also pleases the palate with a variety of flavors and textures. One quarter of the plate should feature whole grains, such as brown rice, quinoa, whole wheat bread, or oatmeal. Whole grains are rich in fiber and nutrients, including B vitamins, antioxidants, and trace minerals like iron, zinc, and magnesium. They provide sustained energy and contribute to digestive health, which is essential for maintaining a balanced diet and supporting the body's overall function. The remaining quarter is reserved for lean protein sources, crucial for building and repairing tissues and maintaining muscle strength. This includes fish, poultry, beans, and nuts, which offer high-quality protein and heart-healthy fats. Incorporating a variety of protein sources can enhance the meal's flavor and nutritional profile, providing essential amino acids and nutrients that support the body's health and well-being. Dairy or dairy alternatives also play a role in the DASH diet, providing calcium, vitamin D, and other essential nutrients for bone health. Opt for low-fat or fat-free options like milk, yogurt, or fortified plant-based alternatives to keep the meal balanced and in line with DASH guidelines. When it comes to portion sizes, the key is moderation. Serving sizes can vary depending on individual needs and activity levels, but general guidelines suggest filling half the plate with fruits and vegetables, one quarter with whole grains, and one quarter with lean proteins. This not only ensures a variety of nutrients but also helps control calories, an important factor in weight management and overall health. Understanding portion sizes is crucial in maintaining this balance. A common method is using your hand as a guide: a fist for vegetables, a palm-sized serving for proteins, a cupped hand for grains, and a thumb-sized portion for fats. This method helps gauge appropriate portions without the need for measuring cups or scales, making it easier to maintain a balanced diet even when dining out or eating on the go. Creating a balanced DASH plate is an art and science, blending the principles of nutrition with the pleasures of eating. It's about enjoying a variety of foods that nourish the body and delight the senses, while also managing portions to support health goals. Each meal is an opportunity to celebrate the rich diversity of nutritious foods available, creating a culinary experience that is both satisfying and healthful.

CHAPTER 3: BREAKFAST DELIGHTS
3.1 HEARTY WHOLE-GRAIN PANCAKES

1. OATMEAL BANANA PANCAKES

P.T.: 10 min

C.T.: 15 min

M.C.: Griddling

SERVINGS: 4

INGR.:

1 cup rolled oats

2 ripe bananas, mashed

2 large eggs

½ cup low-fat milk

1 tsp baking powder

1 tsp vanilla extract

¼ tsp salt

Cooking spray or a little olive oil, for the griddle

PROCEDURE:

In a blender, combine the rolled oats, mashed bananas, eggs, low-fat milk, baking powder, vanilla extract, and salt. Blend until smooth.

Heat a griddle or non-stick pan over medium heat and lightly coat with cooking spray or olive oil.

Pour about ¼ cup of the batter for each pancake onto the griddle. Cook until bubbles appear on the surface, then flip and cook until golden brown on the other side, about 2-3 minutes per side.

Serve warm with your choice of toppings, such as fresh fruit or a drizzle of honey.

TIPS:

Ensure the griddle is at the right temperature before pouring the batter to get evenly cooked pancakes.

Adding a pinch of cinnamon to the batter can enhance the flavor.

N.V.: Calories: 210, Fat: 4g, Carbs: 38g, Protein: 8g, Sugar: 10g

2. WHOLE WHEAT BLUEBERRY PANCAKES

P.T.: 15 min

C.T.: 20 min

M.C.: Griddling

SERVINGS: 4

INGR.:

1½ cups whole wheat flour

1 Tbsp sugar

2 tsp baking powder

½ tsp salt

1 cup low-fat milk

1 large egg

3 Tbsp unsweetened applesauce

1 tsp vanilla extract

1 cup fresh blueberries

Cooking spray or a little olive oil, for the griddle

PROCEDURE:

In a large bowl, whisk together the whole wheat flour, sugar, baking powder, and salt.

In another bowl, mix the milk, egg,

applesauce, and vanilla extract until well combined.

Add the wet ingredients to the dry ingredients and stir until just combined. Fold in the blueberries gently.

Heat a griddle or non-stick pan over medium heat and lightly coat with cooking spray or olive oil.

Pour about ¼ cup of the batter for each pancake onto the griddle. Cook until the edges are set and bubbles appear on the surface, then flip and cook until golden brown on the other side, about 3-4 minutes per side.

Serve hot with a light drizzle of maple syrup or fresh blueberries on top.

TIPS:

Do not overmix the batter to keep the pancakes fluffy.

If blueberries are out of season, frozen ones can be used but ensure they are thawed and well-drained.

N.V.: Calories: 230, Fat: 3g, Carbs: 45g, Protein: 9g, Sugar: 12g

3. BUCKWHEAT AND ALMOND PANCAKES

P.T.: 15 min

C.T.: 15 min

M.C.: Griddling

SERVINGS: 4

INGR.:

1 cup buckwheat flour

½ cup ground almonds

2 tsp baking powder

¼ tsp salt

1 cup low-fat milk

2 large eggs

2 Tbsp honey

1 tsp almond extract

Cooking spray or a little olive oil, for the griddle

PROCEDURE:

In a large bowl, combine buckwheat flour, ground almonds, baking powder, and salt.

In a separate bowl, whisk together the milk, eggs, honey, and almond extract until smooth.

Gradually add the wet ingredients to the dry ingredients, stirring until just combined.

Heat a griddle or non-stick pan over medium heat and lightly coat with cooking spray or olive oil.

Pour about ¼ cup of the batter for each pancake onto the griddle. Cook until bubbles form on the surface, then flip and cook until browned on the other side, approximately 3 minutes per side.

Serve warm with a dollop of Greek yogurt or fresh berries.

TIPS:

Buckwheat flour gives a hearty, nutty flavor to the pancakes, complemented by the almond. Be careful not to overcook, as buckwheat can dry out quickly.

N.V.: Calories: 275, Fat: 10g, Carbs: 38g, Protein: 11g, Sugar: 12g

---

4. QUINOA AND APPLE PANCAKES

P.T.: 20 min

C.T.: 15 min

M.C.: Griddling

SERVINGS: 4

INGR.:

1 cup cooked quinoa

1 cup whole wheat flour

2 tsp baking powder

½ tsp cinnamon

¼ tsp nutmeg

1 cup low-fat milk

2 large eggs

2 Tbsp maple syrup

1 large apple, grated

Cooking spray or a little olive oil, for the griddle

PROCEDURE:

In a large bowl, mix the cooked quinoa, whole wheat flour, baking powder, cinnamon, and nutmeg.

In another bowl, whisk together the milk, eggs, and maple syrup. Stir in the grated apple.

Combine the wet ingredients with the dry ingredients, mixing until just blended.

Heat a griddle or non-stick pan over medium heat and lightly coat with cooking spray or olive oil.

Scoop about ¼ cup of the batter for each pancake onto the griddle. Cook until golden brown on both sides, approximately 4 minutes per side.

Serve warm with a sprinkle of cinnamon and a side of apple compote.

TIPS:

Quinoa adds a wonderful texture and protein boost to the pancakes.

Ensure the griddle is not too hot to prevent the outside from burning before the inside is cooked.

N.V.: Calories: 250, Fat: 4g, Carbs: 43g, Protein: 10g, Sugar: 15g

---

5. MULTI-GRAIN YOGURT PANCAKES

P.T.: 15 min

C.T.: 20 min

M.C.: Griddling

SERVINGS: 4

INGR.:

½ cup whole wheat flour

½ cup rolled oats

½ cup barley flour

2 tsp baking powder

½ tsp salt

1 cup low-fat Greek yogurt

½ cup low-fat milk

2 large eggs

1 Tbsp honey

Cooking spray or a little olive oil, for the griddle

PROCEDURE:

In a large bowl, combine the whole wheat flour, rolled oats, barley flour, baking powder, and salt.

In another bowl, whisk together the Greek yogurt, milk, eggs, and honey until smooth.

Mix the wet ingredients into the dry ingredients until just combined.

Heat a griddle or non-stick pan over medium heat and lightly coat with cooking spray or olive oil.

Pour about ¼ cup of batter for each pancake onto the griddle. Cook until the edges are dry and bubbles form on the surface, then flip and cook until golden brown, about 3-4 minutes per side.

Serve hot with a drizzle of honey or fresh fruit on top.

TIPS:

The combination of grains and yogurt creates a tender texture and tangy flavor.

Avoid overmixing the batter to keep the pancakes light and fluffy.

N.V.: Calories: 280, Fat: 5g, Carbs: 48g, Protein: 14g, Sugar: 10g

---

6. RYE AND WALNUT PANCAKES

P.T.: 15 min

C.T.: 15 min

M.C.: Griddling

SERVINGS: 4

INGR.:

1 cup rye flour

½ cup chopped walnuts

2 tsp baking powder

¼ tsp salt

1 cup low-fat milk

2 large eggs

2 Tbsp maple syrup

Cooking spray or a little olive oil, for the griddle

PROCEDURE:

In a bowl, mix the rye flour, chopped walnuts, baking powder, and salt.

In another bowl, whisk together the milk, eggs, and maple syrup.

Combine the wet and dry ingredients, stirring until just blended.

Heat a griddle or non-stick pan over medium heat and lightly coat with cooking spray or olive oil.

Pour about ¼ cup of the batter for each pancake onto the griddle. Cook until the pancakes are golden brown on both sides, about 3 minutes per side.

Serve warm, topped with additional walnuts and a drizzle of maple syrup.

TIPS:

Rye flour gives a deep, hearty flavor to the pancakes, complemented by the texture of the walnuts.

These pancakes pair well with fruit preserves or a dollop of sour cream for added richness.

N.V.: Calories: 290, Fat: 15g, Carbs: 32g, Protein: 9g, Sugar: 9g

3.2 SPINACH AND MUSHROOM BREAKFAST SKILLET

1. CLASSIC SPINACH AND MUSHROOM BREAKFAST SKILLET

P.T.: 10 min

C.T.: 20 min

M.C.: Sautéing

SERVINGS: 4

INGR.:

1 Tbsp olive oil

1 lb fresh mushrooms, sliced

4 cups fresh spinach

4 large eggs

2 cloves garlic, minced

Salt and pepper to taste

½ tsp red pepper flakes (optional)

PROCEDURE:

Heat the olive oil in a large skillet over medium heat. Add the sliced mushrooms and sauté until they begin to brown, about 5-7 minutes.

Add the minced garlic and red pepper flakes, if using, and cook for another minute until fragrant.

Stir in the spinach and cook until just wilted, about 2-3 minutes.

Make four wells in the mixture and crack an egg into each. Cover and cook until the eggs are set to your liking, about 5-8 minutes.

Season with salt and pepper to taste, and serve hot directly from the skillet.

TIPS:

For an extra flavor boost, sprinkle some grated Parmesan cheese over the skillet just before serving.

Keep the heat on medium to avoid burning the garlic.

N.V.: Calories: 200, Fat: 12g, Carbs: 6g, Protein: 14g, Sugar: 2g

2. MEDITERRANEAN SPINACH AND MUSHROOM SKILLET

P.T.: 15 min

C.T.: 20 min

M.C.: Sautéing

SERVINGS: 4

INGR.:

1 Tbsp olive oil

1 lb fresh mushrooms, sliced

4 cups fresh spinach

1 small onion, diced

2 tomatoes, diced

1/2 cup crumbled feta cheese

4 large eggs

1 tsp dried oregano

Salt and pepper to taste

PROCEDURE:

Heat olive oil in a skillet over medium heat. Add onions and sauté until translucent, about 5 minutes.

Add the mushrooms and cook until they release their moisture and brown slightly, about 8 minutes.

Stir in the tomatoes and oregano, cooking until the tomatoes soften, about 3 minutes.

Add the spinach and cook until it wilts, about 2-3 minutes.

Sprinkle feta cheese over the top, then crack the eggs over the skillet. Cover and cook until the eggs are set, approximately 5-7 minutes.

Season with salt and pepper, and serve warm.

TIPS:

Drizzle a little lemon juice over the skillet before serving for a refreshing zest.

Add sliced black olives for an extra Mediterranean touch.

N.V.: Calories: 250, Fat: 16g, Carbs: 10g, Protein: 17g, Sugar: 4g

3. CHEESY SPINACH AND MUSHROOM SKILLET

P.T.: 10 min

C.T.: 15 min

M.C.: Sautéing

SERVINGS: 4

INGR.:

1 Tbsp olive oil

1 lb fresh mushrooms, sliced

4 cups fresh spinach

4 large eggs

1 cup shredded low-fat cheddar cheese

Salt and pepper to taste

PROCEDURE:

Heat the olive oil in a large skillet over medium heat. Add the mushrooms and sauté until they are golden brown, about 6-8 minutes.

Add the spinach to the skillet and cook until wilted, approximately 2 minutes.

Sprinkle the shredded cheese over the mushroom and spinach mixture.

Carefully crack the eggs on top of the cheese layer, season with salt and pepper, and cover the skillet.

Cook until the eggs are set to your desired doneness, about 5-7 minutes.

Serve immediately, ensuring each portion has an egg and a generous serving of the cheesy spinach and mushroom mixture.

TIPS:

Avoid over-stirring once the eggs are added to keep them intact.

For a melty and golden top, briefly place the skillet under a broiler.

N.V.: Calories: 240, Fat: 16g, Carbs: 7g, Protein: 19g, Sugar: 3g

4. SPINACH AND MUSHROOM QUINOA SKILLET

P.T.: 15 min

C.T.: 25 min

M.C.: Sautéing and simmering

SERVINGS: 4

INGR.:

1 Tbsp olive oil

1 lb fresh mushrooms, sliced

1 cup quinoa, rinsed

2 cups vegetable broth

4 cups fresh spinach

4 large eggs

Salt and pepper to taste

PROCEDURE:

Heat olive oil in a large skillet over medium heat. Add the mushrooms and sauté until they are browned, about 8 minutes.

Stir in the quinoa and vegetable broth, bringing the mixture to a boil.

Reduce heat to low, cover, and simmer for 15 minutes, or until the quinoa is cooked through.

Stir in the spinach and cook until just wilted, about 2 minutes.

Make four wells in the quinoa mixture and crack an egg into each. Season with salt and pepper.

Cover and cook until the eggs are set to your liking, about 5-7 minutes.

Serve hot from the skillet.

TIPS:

Ensure the quinoa is thoroughly rinsed to remove its natural coating, which can be bitter.

Add a splash of lemon juice or a sprinkle of parmesan for an extra flavor boost.

N.V.: Calories: 350, Fat: 15g, Carbs: 35g, Protein: 20g, Sugar: 2g

3.3 BANANA AND WALNUT OATMEAL

1. CLASSIC BANANA AND WALNUT OATMEAL

P.T.: 5 min

C.T.: 10 min

M.C.: Stovetop

SERVINGS: 2

INGR.:

1 cup rolled oats

2 cups water

1 ripe banana, mashed

1/4 cup walnuts, chopped

1 Tbsp honey (optional)

1/2 tsp ground cinnamon

1/4 tsp salt

PROCEDURE:

In a medium saucepan, bring water to a boil.

Add oats and salt, reduce heat to low, and simmer for 5-7 minutes, stirring occasionally.

Stir in mashed banana, walnuts, honey (if using), and cinnamon.

Cook for an additional 2-3 minutes, until the oats are creamy and the banana is well incorporated.

Serve hot, topped with a few extra walnuts and a drizzle of honey if desired.

TIPS:

For extra creaminess, replace half the water with milk or a milk alternative.

Add a handful of fresh berries for added flavor and nutrients.

2. BANANA WALNUT OVERNIGHT OATS

P.T.: 10 min

C.T.: None (Overnight soaking)

M.C.: No-cook

SERVINGS: 2

INGR.:

1 cup rolled oats

1 cup milk or milk alternative

1 ripe banana, mashed

1/4 cup walnuts, chopped

1 Tbsp chia seeds

1 Tbsp maple syrup

1/2 tsp vanilla extract

1/2 tsp ground cinnamon

PROCEDURE:

In a large jar or container, combine oats, milk, mashed banana, walnuts, chia seeds, maple syrup, vanilla extract, and cinnamon. Stir well to ensure all ingredients are evenly distributed.

Cover and refrigerate overnight or for at least 6 hours.

In the morning, give the oats a good stir and add a splash of milk if needed to achieve your desired consistency.

Serve cold or heat in the microwave for a warm option. Top with additional banana slices and walnuts if desired.

TIPS:

Use a ripe banana for natural sweetness, reducing the need for added sweeteners.

For a protein boost, stir in a scoop of your favorite protein powder before refrigerating.

N.V.: Calories: 320, Fat: 12g, Carbs: 50g, Protein: 8g, Sugar: 15g

3. BANANA WALNUT BAKED OATMEAL

P.T.: 10 min

C.T.: 30 min

M.C.: Baking

SERVINGS: 4

INGR.:

2 cups rolled oats

1 tsp baking powder

1/2 tsp salt

1 tsp ground cinnamon

1/4 tsp ground nutmeg

2 ripe bananas, mashed

2 cups milk or milk alternative

1/4 cup walnuts, chopped

2 Tbsp maple syrup

1 tsp vanilla extract

PROCEDURE:

Preheat oven to 375°F (190°C).

In a large bowl, mix together oats, baking powder, salt, cinnamon, and nutmeg.

In another bowl, combine mashed bananas, milk, walnuts, maple syrup, and vanilla extract.

Add the wet ingredients to the dry ingredients and mix until well combined.

Pour the mixture into a greased baking dish.

Bake for 25-30 minutes, until the top is golden brown and the oatmeal is set.

Let cool for a few minutes before serving. Slice and serve warm.

TIPS:

Serve with a dollop of yogurt or a splash of milk.

This baked oatmeal can be stored in the refrigerator for up to 5 days and reheated as needed.

N.V.: Calories: 280, Fat: 8g, Carbs: 45g, Protein: 7g, Sugar: 12g

---

4. BANANA WALNUT OATMEAL SMOOTHIE

P.T.: 5 min

C.T.: None

M.C.: Blending

SERVINGS: 1

INGR.:

1/2 cup rolled oats

1 ripe banana

1/4 cup walnuts

1 cup milk or milk alternative

1 Tbsp honey or maple syrup

1/2 tsp ground cinnamon

1/2 tsp vanilla extract

1 cup ice cubes

PROCEDURE:

Add oats to a blender and pulse until finely ground.

Add banana, walnuts, milk, honey or maple syrup, cinnamon, vanilla extract, and ice cubes.

Blend until smooth and creamy.

Pour into a glass and serve immediately.

TIPS:

For a thicker smoothie, add a spoonful of Greek yogurt.

Use frozen banana slices to make the smoothie even colder and creamier.

N.V.: Calories: 350, Fat: 12g, Carbs: 55g, Protein: 7g, Sugar: 18g

---

5. BANANA WALNUT OATMEAL MUFFINS

P.T.: 15 min

C.T.: 20 min

M.C.: Baking

SERVINGS: 12 muffins

INGR.:

1 1/2 cups rolled oats

1 cup whole wheat flour

1 tsp baking powder

1/2 tsp baking soda

1/2 tsp salt

1 tsp ground cinnamon

2 ripe bananas, mashed

1/2 cup honey

1/4 cup Greek yogurt

2 eggs

1/4 cup milk or milk alternative

1/4 cup walnuts, chopped

PROCEDURE:

Preheat oven to 350°F (175°C).

In a large bowl, mix together oats, flour, baking powder, baking soda, salt, and cinnamon.

In another bowl, combine mashed bananas, honey, Greek yogurt, eggs, and milk.

Add the wet ingredients to the dry ingredients and mix until just combined.

Fold in the chopped walnuts.

Divide the batter evenly among a greased or lined muffin tin.

Bake for 18-20 minutes, until a toothpick inserted into the center of a muffin comes out clean.

Let cool in the tin for 5 minutes, then transfer to a wire rack to cool completely.

TIPS:

For extra crunch, sprinkle a few chopped walnuts on top of each muffin before baking.

These muffins can be frozen for up to 3 months; simply reheat in the microwave for a quick breakfast.

N.V.: Calories: 190, Fat: 5g, Carbs: 33g, Protein: 4g, Sugar: 14g

CHAPTER 4: LIGHT LUNCHES

4.1 QUINOA SALAD WITH MIXED GREENS

1. CLASSIC QUINOA AND MIXED GREENS SALAD

P.T.: 15 min

C.T.: 20 min

M.C.: Boiling

SERVINGS: 4

INGR.:

1 cup quinoa, rinsed

2 cups water

4 cups mixed greens (like spinach, arugula, and romaine)

1 cucumber, diced

1 red bell pepper, diced

¼ cup red onion, finely chopped

¼ cup feta cheese, crumbled

¼ cup balsamic vinaigrette dressing

Salt and pepper to taste

PROCEDURE:

In a medium saucepan, bring 2 cups of water to a boil. Add the quinoa, reduce heat to low, cover, and simmer for 15-20 minutes or until the quinoa is tender and water is absorbed.

Let the quinoa cool to room temperature, then fluff with a fork.

In a large bowl, combine the cooked quinoa, mixed greens, cucumber, red bell pepper, and red onion.

Toss the salad with balsamic vinaigrette dressing, then sprinkle with feta cheese.

Season with salt and pepper, and serve chilled or at room temperature.

TIPS:

To add a crunch, top the salad with toasted nuts or seeds.

For a zestier flavor, include a squeeze of fresh lemon juice in the dressing.

N.V.: Calories: 250, Fat: 8g, Carbs: 35g, Protein: 10g, Sugar: 4g

2. MEDITERRANEAN QUINOA AND GREENS SALAD

P.T.: 20 min

C.T.: 20 min

M.C.: Boiling

SERVINGS: 4

INGR.:

1 cup quinoa, rinsed

2 cups vegetable broth

4 cups mixed greens (such as baby spinach and arugula)

1 cup cherry tomatoes, halved

½ cup cucumber, diced

½ cup Kalamata olives, pitted and halved

½ cup artichoke hearts, quartered

¼ cup crumbled feta cheese

1 lemon, juiced

3 Tbsp olive oil

1 tsp dried oregano

Salt and pepper to taste

PROCEDURE:

Cook quinoa in vegetable broth according to

package instructions, then let it cool.

In a large salad bowl, combine the mixed greens, cherry tomatoes, cucumber, olives, and artichoke hearts. In a small bowl, whisk together lemon juice, olive oil, oregano, salt, and pepper to make the dressing. Add the cooled quinoa to the salad bowl and toss with the dressing. Sprinkle feta cheese over the top before serving.

TIPS:

Enhance the Mediterranean flavor with a sprinkle of fresh herbs like basil or parsley. For added protein, include grilled chicken or chickpeas.

N.V.: Calories: 300, Fat: 15g, Carbs: 35g, Protein: 8g, Sugar: 5g

3. ASIAN-STYLE QUINOA AND GREENS SALAD

P.T.: 20 min

C.T.: 20 min

M.C.: Boiling

SERVINGS: 4

INGR.:

1 cup quinoa, rinsed

2 cups water

4 cups mixed greens (like baby bok choy, spinach, and kale)

1 carrot, julienned

1 red bell pepper, thinly sliced

½ cup edamame, shelled and cooked

2 Tbsp sesame seeds

For the dressing:

2 Tbsp soy sauce

1 Tbsp sesame oil

1 Tbsp rice vinegar

1 tsp honey

1 garlic clove, minced

1 tsp fresh ginger, grated

PROCEDURE:

Cook quinoa in water according to package instructions, then let it cool to room temperature. In a large bowl, combine mixed greens, carrot, red bell pepper, and edamame. In a small bowl, whisk together soy sauce, sesame oil, rice vinegar, honey, garlic, and ginger to create the dressing. Toss the cooled quinoa with the salad mixture, then drizzle with the dressing and mix well. Garnish with sesame seeds before serving.

TIPS:

Add grilled tofu or chicken for extra protein. Make sure the quinoa is completely cool before mixing with the greens to keep them crisp.

N.V.: Calories: 280, Fat: 10g, Carbs: 36g, Protein: 12g, Sugar: 6g

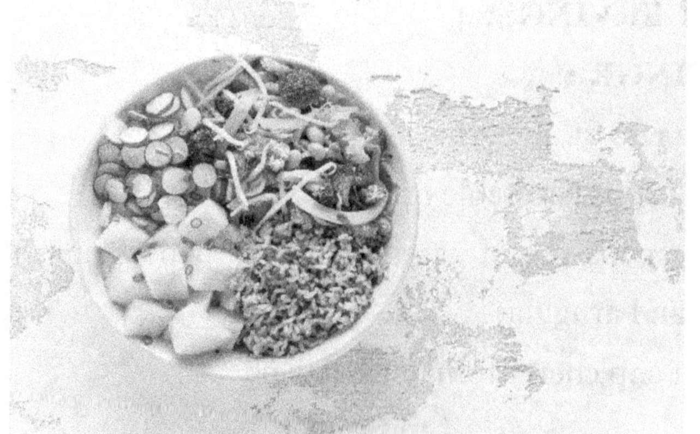

P.T.: 15 min

C.T.: 20 min

M.C.: Boiling

SERVINGS: 4

INGR.:

1 cup quinoa, rinsed

2 cups water

4 cups mixed greens (such as arugula and romaine)

1 ripe avocado, diced

½ cup cherry tomatoes, halved

¼ cup red onion, thinly sliced

2 Tbsp pumpkin seeds

For the dressing:

2 Tbsp lime juice

3 Tbsp olive oil

1 tsp honey

Salt and pepper to taste

PROCEDURE:

Cook quinoa in water according to package instructions, then let it cool.

In a large bowl, combine mixed greens, avocado, cherry tomatoes, and red onion.

In a small bowl, whisk together lime juice, olive oil, honey, salt, and pepper to make the dressing.

Add the cooled quinoa to the salad bowl, toss with the dressing, and mix well.

Sprinkle with pumpkin seeds before serving.

TIPS:

The avocado adds creaminess to the salad, so it's best consumed fresh to prevent browning.

For a crunch, add crumbled baked tortilla chips on top.

N.V.: Calories: 320, Fat: 18g, Carbs: 34g, Protein: 8g, Sugar: 5g

P.T.: 20 min

C.T.: 20 min

M.C.: Boiling

SERVINGS: 4

INGR.:

1 cup quinoa, rinsed

2 cups water

4 cups mixed greens (such as spinach and romaine)

½ cup cucumber, diced

½ cup cherry tomatoes, halved

¼ cup Kalamata olives, pitted and halved

¼ cup red onion, thinly sliced

½ cup feta cheese, crumbled

For the dressing:

3 Tbsp olive oil

1 Tbsp red wine vinegar

1 tsp dried oregano

Salt and pepper to taste

PROCEDURE:

Cook quinoa in water according to package instructions, then let it cool.

In a large salad bowl, combine mixed greens, cucumber, cherry tomatoes, olives, and red onion.

For the dressing, whisk together olive oil, red

wine vinegar, oregano, salt, and pepper in a small bowl.

Toss the cooled quinoa and salad mixture with the dressing, then crumble feta cheese over the top before serving.

TIPS:

For an authentic Greek flavor, add a sprinkle of fresh herbs like dill or parsley.

Drizzle a little lemon juice over the salad for added zest.

N.V.: Calories: 300, Fat: 16g, Carbs: 30g, Protein: 10g, Sugar: 4g

---

6. ROASTED VEGETABLE QUINOA AND GREENS SALAD

P.T.: 20 min

C.T.: 30 min

M.C.: Roasting and boiling

SERVINGS: 4

INGR.:

1 cup quinoa, rinsed

2 cups water

2 cups mixed greens (like kale and spinach)

1 red bell pepper, chopped

1 zucchini, chopped

1 yellow squash, chopped

1 eggplant, chopped

3 Tbsp olive oil, divided

Salt and pepper to taste

2 Tbsp balsamic vinegar

PROCEDURE:

Preheat the oven to 400°F (200°C). Toss the chopped vegetables with 2 Tbsp olive oil, salt, and pepper, then spread on a baking sheet.

Roast for 25-30 minutes, or until vegetables are tender and lightly browned. Meanwhile, cook quinoa in water according to package instructions, then let it cool. In a large bowl, combine roasted vegetables, cooled quinoa, and mixed greens. Drizzle with remaining 1 Tbsp olive oil and balsamic vinegar, toss to combine, and season with additional salt and pepper if needed. Serve warm or at room temperature.

TIPS:

Experiment with different seasonal vegetables for variety throughout the year. For added protein, toss in some chickpeas or grilled chicken.

N.V.: Calories: 330, Fat: 15g, Carbs: 42g, Protein: 10g, Sugar: 7g

4.2 TURKEY AND AVOCADO WRAP

1. CLASSIC TURKEY AND AVOCADO WRAP

P.T.: 10 min

C.T.: 0 min

M.C.: No cook

SERVINGS: 4

INGR.:

4 whole wheat tortillas

8 slices turkey breast

2 ripe avocados, sliced

2 cups mixed greens

1 tomato, sliced

1 small red onion, thinly sliced

4 Tbsp low-fat Greek yogurt

Salt and pepper to taste

PROCEDURE:

Lay out the tortillas on a flat surface.

Spread each tortilla with 1 tablespoon of Greek yogurt.

Layer the turkey slices, avocado, mixed greens, tomato, and red onion on top of each tortilla.

Season with salt and pepper.

Roll the tortillas tightly, tucking in the sides as you go, to form the wraps.

Cut in half and serve immediately.

TIPS:

For a gluten-free option, use gluten-free tortillas.

Add a sprinkle of paprika or cumin for an extra flavor kick.

N.V.: Calories: 350, Fat: 15g, Carbs: 35g, Protein: 20g, Sugar: 5g

---

2. SPICY TURKEY AND AVOCADO WRAP

P.T.: 10 min

C.T.: 0 min

M.C.: No cook

SERVINGS: 4

INGR.:

4 whole wheat tortillas

8 slices turkey breast

2 ripe avocados, mashed

2 cups baby spinach

½ cup cucumber, thinly sliced

1 small jalapeño, seeded and finely chopped

4 Tbsp low-fat sour cream

1 lime, juiced

Salt and pepper to taste

PROCEDURE:

In a small bowl, mix the mashed avocado with lime juice, jalapeño, salt, and pepper.

Spread each tortilla with a tablespoon of sour cream.

Add a layer of turkey slices, then top with the spicy avocado mixture, spinach, and cucumber slices.

Roll the tortillas tightly, tucking in the sides to secure the filling.

Cut the wraps in half and serve.

TIPS:

Adjust the amount of jalapeño according to your spice preference.

A drizzle of hot sauce can intensify the flavor for those who prefer an extra kick.

N.V.: Calories: 360, Fat: 16g, Carbs: 36g, Protein: 22g, Sugar: 4g

P.T.: 15 min

C.T.: 0 min

M.C.: No cook

SERVINGS: 4

INGR.:

4 whole grain tortillas

8 slices turkey breast

2 ripe avocados, sliced

1 cup arugula

½ cup sun-dried tomatoes, chopped

¼ cup goat cheese, crumbled

2 Tbsp pesto sauce

Salt and pepper to taste

PROCEDURE:

Spread each tortilla with a layer of pesto sauce.

Place two slices of turkey breast on each tortilla, followed by avocado slices, arugula, sun-dried tomatoes, and crumbled goat cheese.

Season with salt and pepper.

Roll up the tortillas tightly, ensuring the filling is evenly distributed.

Cut each wrap in half and serve immediately.

TIPS:

For a lower-fat option, replace goat cheese with a light cream cheese.

Ensure the sun-dried tomatoes are not overly oily to prevent the wrap from becoming soggy.

N.V.: Calories: 400, Fat: 20g, Carbs: 40g, Protein: 24g, Sugar: 6g

4.3 HOMEMADE VEGETABLE SOUP

P.T.: 15 min

C.T.: 30 min

M.C.: Simmering

SERVINGS: 4

INGR.:

1 Tbsp olive oil

1 onion, chopped

2 carrots, peeled and diced

2 celery stalks, diced

1 zucchini, diced

2 garlic cloves, minced

4 cups vegetable broth

2 tomatoes, diced

1 cup green beans, trimmed and cut into 1-inch pieces

1 tsp dried basil

1 tsp dried oregano

Salt and pepper to taste

PROCEDURE:

Heat olive oil in a large pot over medium heat.

Add onion, carrots, and celery, sautéing until softened, about 5 minutes.

Stir in garlic and zucchini, cooking for another 2 minutes.

Add vegetable broth, tomatoes, green beans, basil, and oregano. Bring to a boil.

Reduce heat and simmer, covered, for 20 minutes or until vegetables are tender. Season with salt and pepper to taste. Serve hot.

TIPS:

Add a can of drained and rinsed white beans for extra protein and fiber.

Serve with a sprinkle of grated Parmesan cheese for added flavor.

N.V.: Calories: 120, Fat: 3.5g, Carbs: 20g, Protein: 4g, Sugar: 8g

---

2. SPICY TOMATO AND RED PEPPER SOUP

P.T.: 10 min

C.T.: 20 min

M.C.: Blending and simmering

SERVINGS: 4

INGR.:

1 Tbsp olive oil

1 onion, chopped

2 red bell peppers, chopped

2 garlic cloves, minced

1 tsp smoked paprika

1 tsp red pepper flakes (optional)

4 cups tomato puree

2 cups vegetable broth

Salt and pepper to taste

Fresh basil leaves for garnish

PROCEDURE:

In a large pot, heat olive oil over medium heat. Add onion and bell peppers, cooking until softened, about 5 minutes.

Add garlic, smoked paprika, and red pepper flakes, cooking for another minute.

Stir in tomato puree and vegetable broth, bring to a simmer, and cook for 15 minutes.

Use an immersion blender to puree the soup until smooth (or carefully transfer to a blender).

Season with salt and pepper, and serve garnished with fresh basil leaves.

TIPS:

For a creamier texture, add a splash of coconut milk or light cream before serving.

Adjust the heat level by increasing or decreasing the amount of red pepper flakes.

N.V.: Calories: 150, Fat: 4g, Carbs: 25g, Protein: 4g, Sugar: 15g

---

3. HEARTY LENTIL AND VEGETABLE SOUP

P.T.: 15 min

C.T.: 45 min

M.C.: Simmering

SERVINGS: 4

INGR.:

1 Tbsp olive oil

1 onion, diced

2 carrots, peeled and diced

2 celery stalks, diced

2 garlic cloves, minced

1 cup lentils, rinsed

4 cups vegetable broth

2 cups water

1 tsp ground cumin

1 tsp dried thyme

1 bay leaf

Salt and pepper to taste

2 cups chopped kale or spinach

PROCEDURE:

Heat olive oil in a large pot over medium heat.

Add onion, carrots, and celery, and sauté until softened, about 5 minutes.

Stir in garlic, lentils, cumin, thyme, and bay leaf, cooking for 1 minute.

Add vegetable broth and water. Bring to a boil, then reduce heat and simmer, partially covered, for 30 minutes or until lentils are tender.

Add kale or spinach and cook until wilted, about 5 minutes. Remove the bay leaf, season with salt and pepper, and serve hot.

TIPS:

Soaking lentils overnight can reduce cooking time and improve digestibility.

Add a splash of lemon juice before serving for a fresh, tangy flavor.

N.V.: Calories: 240, Fat: 5g, Carbs: 38g, Protein: 14g, Sugar: 6g

---

4. CREAMY BROCCOLI AND POTATO SOUP

P.T.: 15 min

C.T.: 30 min

M.C.: Simmering and blending

SERVINGS: 4

INGR.:

1 Tbsp olive oil

1 onion, chopped

2 cloves garlic, minced

2 large potatoes, peeled and cubed

4 cups broccoli florets

4 cups vegetable broth

Salt and pepper to taste

½ cup low-fat milk or almond milk

Chopped chives for garnish

PROCEDURE:

In a large pot, heat olive oil over medium heat. Sauté onion and garlic until translucent, about 5 minutes.

Add potatoes, broccoli, and vegetable broth. Bring to a boil, then reduce heat and simmer until the potatoes are tender, about 20 minutes.

Use an immersion blender to puree the soup until smooth.

Stir in the milk, season with salt and pepper, and heat through.

Serve garnished with chopped chives.

TIPS:

For a thicker soup, reserve some of the cooked broccoli and potatoes to add texture after blending.

Nutritional yeast can be added for a cheesy flavor without the dairy.

N.V.: Calories: 200, Fat: 4g, Carbs: 36g, Protein: 8g, Sugar: 6g

P.T.: 15 min

C.T.: 25 min

M.C.: Simmering

SERVINGS: 4

INGR.:

1 Tbsp olive oil

1 onion, chopped

2 cloves garlic, minced

2 cups cauliflower florets

2 carrots, peeled and diced

1 Tbsp curry powder

4 cups vegetable broth

Salt and pepper to taste

Fresh cilantro for garnish

PROCEDURE:

In a large pot, heat olive oil over medium heat. Add onion and garlic, cooking until softened, about 5 minutes.

Stir in cauliflower, carrots, and curry powder, cooking for 2 minutes.

Add vegetable broth, bring to a boil, then reduce heat and simmer until vegetables are tender, about 15-20 minutes.

Puree the soup using an immersion blender until smooth.

Season with salt and pepper, and serve garnished with fresh cilantro.

TIPS:

Adjust the amount of curry powder to suit your taste preferences.

Coconut milk can be added for a creamier texture and a subtle sweetness.

N.V.: Calories: 150, Fat: 5g, Carbs: 22g, Protein: 4g, Sugar: 8g

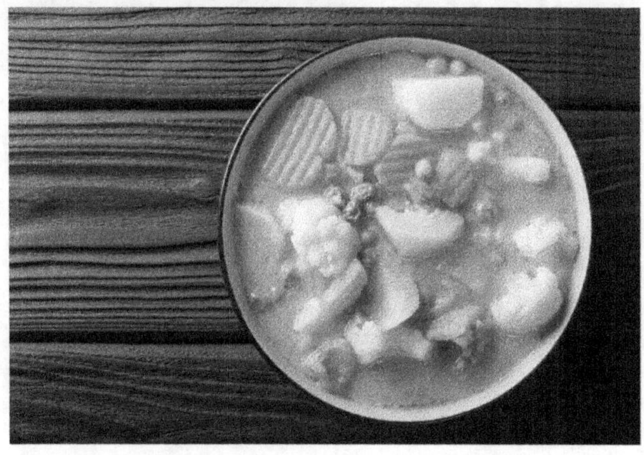

CHAPTER 5: SATISFYING SNACKS
5.1 HUMMUS AND VEGGIE STICKS

1. CLASSIC CHICKPEA HUMMUS WITH ASSORTED VEGGIE STICKS

P.T.: 10 min

C.T.: 0 min

M.C.: Blending

SERVINGS: 4

INGR.:

1 can (15 oz) chickpeas, drained and rinsed

2 Tbsp tahini

2 garlic cloves, minced

2 Tbsp lemon juice

2 Tbsp olive oil

Salt and pepper to taste

Water as needed

Veggie sticks (carrot, cucumber, bell pepper, and celery)

PROCEDURE:

In a food processor, blend chickpeas, tahini, garlic, lemon juice, and olive oil until smooth. Add water as needed to reach the desired consistency. Season with salt and pepper. Serve the hummus with an assortment of fresh veggie sticks.

TIPS:

For a smoother hummus, peel the chickpeas before blending.

Drizzle a bit of olive oil and sprinkle some paprika on top of the hummus before serving for added flavor.

N.V.: Calories: 180, Fat: 10g, Carbs: 18g, Protein: 6g, Sugar: 3g

2. ROASTED RED PEPPER HUMMUS WITH ZUCCHINI STICKS

P.T.: 15 min

C.T.: 0 min

M.C.: Blending

SERVINGS: 4

INGR.:

1 can (15 oz) chickpeas, drained and rinsed

1 roasted red pepper, peeled and seeded

2 Tbsp tahini

1 garlic clove, minced

2 Tbsp lemon juice

1 Tbsp olive oil

Salt and pepper to taste

Zucchini, cut into sticks

PROCEDURE:

Combine chickpeas, roasted red pepper, tahini, garlic, lemon juice, and olive oil in a food processor. Blend until smooth. Season with salt and pepper to taste. Serve with zucchini sticks for dipping.

TIPS:

Roast your own red peppers for a fresher taste, or use jarred roasted red peppers for convenience. Add a pinch of cumin or smoked paprika for a flavor twist.

N.V.: Calories: 190, Fat: 9g, Carbs: 22g, Protein: 7g, Sugar: 4g

P.T.: 15 min

C.T.: 0 min

M.C.: Blending

SERVINGS: 4

INGR.:

1 can (15 oz) chickpeas, drained and rinsed

1 medium beetroot, cooked and peeled

2 Tbsp tahini

1 garlic clove, minced

2 Tbsp lemon juice

2 Tbsp olive oil

Salt and pepper to taste

Cauliflower, cut into florets or sticks

PROCEDURE:

In a food processor, combine chickpeas, beetroot, tahini, garlic, lemon juice, and olive oil. Blend until smooth.

Add salt and pepper to taste, adjusting seasoning as necessary.

Serve the vibrant beetroot hummus with cauliflower sticks for a healthy and colorful snack.

TIPS:

Roast the beetroot before blending to enhance its sweet, earthy flavor.

For a creamier texture, add a little Greek yogurt to the hummus mixture.

N.V.: Calories: 200, Fat: 11g, Carbs: 20g, Protein: 7g, Sugar: 5g

P.T.: 15 min

C.T.: 0 min

M.C.: Blending

SERVINGS: 4

INGR.:

1 can (15 oz) chickpeas, drained and rinsed

1 ripe avocado

2 Tbsp tahini

1 garlic clove, minced

3 Tbsp lime juice

2 Tbsp olive oil

Salt and pepper to taste

Sweet potato, cut into sticks and roasted or raw

PROCEDURE:

Blend chickpeas, avocado, tahini, garlic, lime juice, and olive oil in a food processor until smooth.

Season the hummus with salt and pepper to your liking.

Serve with sweet potato sticks, either raw for crunch or roasted for a softer texture.

TIPS:

The addition of avocado not only adds creaminess but also provides healthy fats and a subtle buttery flavor.

Lime juice enhances the freshness of the hummus and pairs well with the avocado.

N.V.: Calories: 230, Fat: 14g, Carbs: 23g, Protein: 7g, Sugar: 4g

5.2 Fruit and Nut Yogurt Parfaits

1. Mixed Berry and Almond Yogurt Parfait

P.T.: 10 min

C.T.: 0 min

M.C.: Layering

SERVINGS: 4

INGR.:

2 cups low-fat Greek yogurt

1 cup mixed berries (strawberries, blueberries, raspberries)

½ cup granola

¼ cup sliced almonds

2 Tbsp honey

PROCEDURE:

In four glasses or parfait cups, layer the Greek yogurt, mixed berries, and granola.

Repeat the layers until all ingredients are used.

Top each parfait with sliced almonds and drizzle with honey.

TIPS:

For added flavor, mix a teaspoon of vanilla extract into the yogurt before layering.

Fresh berries are preferable, but frozen and thawed berries can be used as an alternative.

N.V.: Calories: 220, Fat: 6g, Carbs: 30g, Protein: 12g, Sugar: 18g

2. Tropical Mango and Coconut Yogurt Parfait

P.T.: 10 min

C.T.: 0 min

M.C.: Layering

SERVINGS: 4

INGR.:

2 cups low-fat Greek yogurt

1 cup fresh mango, diced

½ cup granola

¼ cup shredded coconut, toasted

2 Tbsp agave nectar

PROCEDURE:

Begin by layering Greek yogurt, diced mango, and granola in four parfait glasses.

Repeat the layers, finishing with a layer of yogurt.

Top each parfait with toasted coconut and drizzle with agave nectar.

TIPS:

Ensure the mango is ripe for the best flavor and natural sweetness.

Toasting the coconut enhances its flavor and adds a delightful crunch.

N.V.: Calories: 230, Fat: 7g, Carbs: 32g, Protein: 12g, Sugar: 20g

3. Apple Cinnamon and Walnut Yogurt Parfait

P.T.: 15 min

C.T.: 0 min

M.C.: Layering

SERVINGS: 4

INGR.:

2 cups low-fat Greek yogurt

1 cup apples, diced

½ tsp ground cinnamon

½ cup granola

¼ cup walnuts, chopped

2 Tbsp maple syrup

PROCEDURE:

Mix the diced apples with ground cinnamon in a bowl.

In four parfait glasses, layer the Greek yogurt, cinnamon apples, and granola.

Repeat the layers, finishing with a layer of yogurt.

Top each parfait with chopped walnuts and drizzle with maple syrup.

TIPS:

For a touch of warmth and spice, lightly sauté the apples and cinnamon in a pan before layering.

Choose a tart apple variety, like Granny Smith, for a nice contrast with the sweet yogurt and syrup.

N.V.: Calories: 250, Fat: 8g, Carbs: 34g, Protein: 12g, Sugar: 22g

4. PEAR AND PECAN YOGURT PARFAIT

P.T.: 10 min

C.T.: 0 min

M.C.: Layering

SERVINGS: 4

INGR.:

2 cups low-fat Greek yogurt

1 cup pears, diced

½ cup granola

¼ cup pecans, chopped

2 Tbsp honey

PROCEDURE:

Start by layering Greek yogurt, diced pears, and granola in four parfait glasses.

Repeat the layers, ending with a final layer of yogurt on top.

Garnish each parfait with chopped pecans and a drizzle of honey.

TIPS:

Lightly toss the diced pears in lemon juice to prevent browning and add a zesty flavor.

Toasting the pecans before adding them to the parfait can enhance their nutty taste and add extra crunch.

N.V.: Calories: 240, Fat: 9g, Carbs: 32g, Protein: 11g, Sugar: 20g

5.3 ALMOND AND APRICOT BITES

1. CLASSIC ALMOND AND APRICOT BITES

P.T.: 15 min

C.T.: 0 min

M.C.: No cook

SERVINGS: 12 bites

INGR.:

1 cup dried apricots

½ cup raw almonds

1 Tbsp honey

1 tsp orange zest

¼ cup unsweetened shredded coconut

PROCEDURE:

In a food processor, blend the apricots, almonds, honey, and orange zest until the mixture forms a sticky dough.

Roll the mixture into small bite-sized balls.

Roll each ball in shredded coconut to coat.

Chill in the refrigerator for at least 1 hour before serving.

TIPS:

For a nuttier flavor, lightly toast the almonds before blending.

If the mixture is too sticky, chill it in the refrigerator for 30 minutes before rolling into balls.

N.V.: Calories: 80, Fat: 4g, Carbs: 10g, Protein: 2g, Sugar: 8g

2. CHOCOLATE-DIPPED ALMOND AND APRICOT BITES

P.T.: 20 min

C.T.: 0 min

M.C.: No cook

SERVINGS: 12 bites

INGR.:

1 cup dried apricots

½ cup roasted almonds

2 Tbsp cocoa powder

1 Tbsp honey

½ tsp vanilla extract

100g dark chocolate, melted

PROCEDURE:

In a food processor, blend the apricots, almonds, cocoa powder, honey, and vanilla extract until combined.

Form the mixture into small balls.

Dip each ball into melted dark chocolate, coating half or the entire ball.

Place on a parchment-lined tray and refrigerate until the chocolate sets.

TIPS:

Use high-quality dark chocolate with at least 70% cocoa for added antioxidants.

Keep the bites refrigerated in an airtight container to maintain freshness.

N.V.: Calories: 100, Fat: 6g, Carbs: 12g, Protein: 2g, Sugar: 9g

3. ALMOND AND APRICOT ENERGY BALLS WITH CHIA SEEDS

P.T.: 15 min

C.T.: 0 min

M.C.: No cook

SERVINGS: 12 bites

INGR.:

1 cup dried apricots

½ cup almonds

2 Tbsp chia seeds

1 Tbsp honey

1 tsp lemon zest

¼ cup rolled oats

PROCEDURE:

In a food processor, blend the dried apricots, almonds, chia seeds, honey, and lemon zest until the mixture sticks together.

Transfer to a bowl and stir in the rolled oats until well combined.

Roll the mixture into small balls, about the size of a walnut.

Refrigerate for at least 1 hour to set before serving.

TIPS:

Soak the dried apricots in warm water for 10 minutes before blending if they are too hard. Rolling the balls in extra chia seeds or oats after shaping can add texture and visual appeal.

N.V.: Calories: 90, Fat: 4.5g, Carbs: 11g, Protein: 3g, Sugar: 7g

4. ALMOND, APRICOT, AND COCONUT BLISS BALLS

P.T.: 20 min

C.T.: 0 min

M.C.: No cook

SERVINGS: 12 bites

INGR.:

1 cup dried apricots

½ cup almonds

¼ cup unsweetened shredded coconut, plus extra for rolling

1 Tbsp coconut oil

1 tsp vanilla extract

PROCEDURE:

Process the dried apricots, almonds, shredded coconut, coconut oil, and vanilla extract in a food processor until the mixture forms a sticky dough. Roll the mixture into small, bite-sized balls. Roll each ball in additional shredded coconut to coat. Chill in the refrigerator for at least 1 hour to firm up before serving.

TIPS:

To enhance the coconut flavor, lightly toast the shredded coconut before adding it to the food processor. Keep the bliss balls in an airtight container in the refrigerator to maintain freshness.

N.V.: Calories: 100, Fat: 6g, Carbs: 10g, Protein: 2g, Sugar: 8g

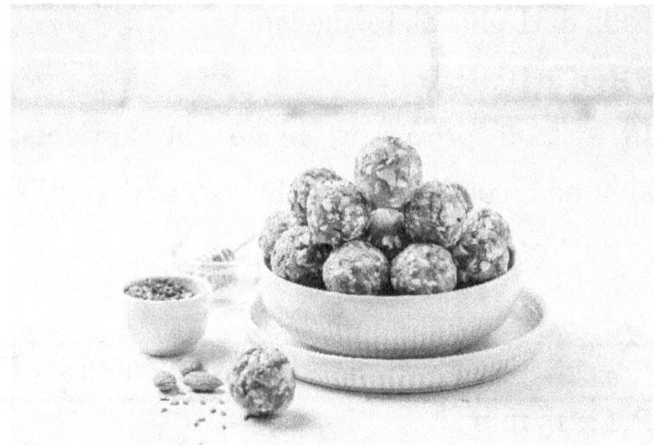

CHAPTER 6: DASH DIET DINNER WINS

6.1 LEMON AND HERB GRILLED CHICKEN

1. CLASSIC LEMON HERB GRILLED CHICKEN

P.T.: 15 min (plus marinating time)

C.T.: 20 min

M.C.: Grilling

SERVINGS: 4

INGR.:

4 boneless, skinless chicken breasts

2 lemons, juiced and zested

2 Tbsp olive oil

3 garlic cloves, minced

1 Tbsp fresh rosemary, chopped

1 Tbsp fresh thyme, chopped

Salt and pepper to taste

PROCEDURE:

In a bowl, whisk together lemon juice, lemon zest, olive oil, garlic, rosemary, thyme, salt, and pepper.

Place chicken breasts in a resealable plastic bag or shallow dish and pour the marinade over them. Ensure all pieces are evenly coated.

Refrigerate and marinate for at least 2 hours, preferably overnight.

Preheat the grill to medium-high heat. Grill chicken breasts for 10 minutes per side or until fully cooked and internal temperature reaches 165°F (74°C).

Let the chicken rest for 5 minutes before slicing and serving.

TIPS:

Marinating the chicken for longer will enhance the flavors and tenderness.

Ensure the grill is hot before adding the chicken to prevent sticking and to achieve nice grill marks.

N.V.: Calories: 240, Fat: 8g, Carbs: 3g, Protein: 36g, Sugar: 1g

2. LEMON GARLIC CHICKEN WITH MEDITERRANEAN HERBS

P.T.: 20 min (plus marinating time)

C.T.: 20 min

M.C.: Grilling

SERVINGS: 4

INGR.:

4 boneless, skinless chicken breasts

2 lemons, juiced

4 garlic cloves, minced

2 Tbsp olive oil

1 tsp dried oregano

1 tsp dried basil

1 tsp dried parsley

Salt and pepper to taste

PROCEDURE:

Combine lemon juice, minced garlic, olive oil, oregano, basil, parsley, salt, and pepper in a bowl to create the marinade.

Marinate the chicken breasts as described in the first recipe, for at least 2 hours or overnight.

Preheat the grill to medium-high and grill the chicken for about 10 minutes on each side or until cooked through.

Rest the chicken for a few minutes before serving.

TIPS:

Adding a pinch of red pepper flakes to the marinade can provide a spicy kick.

Serve with a side of grilled vegetables or a fresh Greek salad for a complete Mediterranean meal.

N.V.: Calories: 250, Fat: 9g, Carbs: 4g, Protein: 36g, Sugar: 1g

---

3. CITRUS HERB CHICKEN PICCATA

P.T.: 15 min

C.T.: 20 min

M.C.: Sautéing

SERVINGS: 4

INGR.:

4 boneless, skinless chicken breasts, pounded to even thickness

1/4 cup whole wheat flour (for dredging)

2 Tbsp olive oil

1/3 cup fresh lemon juice

1/2 cup low-sodium chicken broth

2 Tbsp capers, rinsed

1 Tbsp fresh parsley, chopped

1 lemon, sliced into rounds

Salt (optional) and pepper to taste

DIRECTIONS:

Season the chicken breasts with salt (if using) and pepper, then dredge in whole wheat flour, shaking off the excess.

Heat olive oil in a large skillet over medium-high heat. Add the chicken and cook until golden brown on both sides and cooked through, about 3-4 minutes per side. Remove chicken and set aside.

In the same skillet, add lemon juice, chicken broth, and capers. Bring to a simmer, scraping up any brown bits from the bottom of the pan.

Return the chicken to the skillet and simmer in the sauce for about 5 minutes.

Serve the chicken topped with sauce, garnished with fresh parsley and lemon slices.

TIPS:

For a thicker sauce, you can whisk in a teaspoon of whole wheat flour after adding the chicken broth.

Serve with a side of steamed green beans or asparagus for a complete meal.

N.V.: Calories: 235, Fat: 10g, Carbs: 8g, Protein: 28g, Sugar: 2g

---

4. GRILLED LEMON PEPPER CHICKEN

P.T.: 15 min (plus at least 1 hr for marinating)

C.T.: 14 min

M.C.: Grilling

SERVINGS: 4

INGR.:

4 boneless, skinless chicken breasts

1/4 cup olive oil

1/4 cup lemon juice

1 Tbsp lemon zest

1 Tbsp cracked black pepper

2 cloves garlic, minced

Salt (optional) to taste

DIRECTIONS:

In a small bowl, whisk together olive oil, lemon juice, lemon zest, cracked black pepper, garlic, and salt (if using) to create the marinade.

Place chicken breasts in a resealable plastic bag and pour in the marinade. Seal and shake to coat the chicken evenly. Marinate in the refrigerator for at least 1 hour, preferably longer.

Preheat grill to medium-high heat. Remove chicken from marinade, letting excess drip off.

Grill chicken for 7 minutes on each side, or until it reaches an internal temperature of 165°F (74°C) and is nicely charred.

Let the chicken rest for a few minutes before slicing and serving.

TIPS:

The longer the chicken marinates, the more flavorful it will be. Overnight marinating is recommended for the best result.

Pair with a light quinoa salad or grilled vegetables for a balanced meal.

N.V.: Calories: 220, Fat: 9g, Carbs: 2g, Protein: 31g, Sugar: 0g

6.2 BLACK BEAN AND SWEET POTATO STEW

1. CLASSIC BLACK BEAN AND SWEET POTATO STEW

P.T.: 15 min

C.T.: 30 min

M.C.: Simmering

SERVINGS: 6

INGR.:

2 Tbsp olive oil

1 large onion, diced

2 cloves garlic, minced

2 large sweet potatoes, peeled and cubed

1 red bell pepper, diced

2 cans (15 oz each) black beans, rinsed and drained

1 can (14.5 oz) diced tomatoes

4 cups low-sodium vegetable broth

1 tsp ground cumin

1 tsp smoked paprika

Salt (optional) and pepper to taste

Fresh cilantro, chopped for garnish

DIRECTIONS:

Heat olive oil in a large pot over medium heat.

Add onion and garlic, sauté until soft.

Add sweet potatoes and bell pepper, cook for 5 minutes, stirring occasionally.

Stir in black beans, diced tomatoes, vegetable broth, cumin, and smoked paprika. Season with salt (if using) and pepper.

Bring to a boil, then reduce heat and simmer, covered, for 25 minutes, or until sweet potatoes are tender.

Serve hot, garnished with fresh cilantro.

TIPS:

For a thicker stew, mash some of the sweet potatoes against the side of the pot before serving.

Serve with a side of whole-grain bread for dipping.

N.V.: Calories: 250, Fat: 5g, Carbs: 45g, Protein: 10g, Sugar: 8g

---

2. SPICY CHIPOTLE BLACK BEAN AND SWEET POTATO CHILI

P.T.: 20 min

C.T.: 40 min

M.C.: Simmering

SERVINGS: 6

INGR.:

2 Tbsp olive oil

1 onion, chopped

3 cloves garlic, minced

2 sweet potatoes, peeled and cubed

2 cans (15 oz each) black beans, drained and rinsed

2 chipotle peppers in adobo sauce, finely chopped

1 can (28 oz) crushed tomatoes

3 cups low-sodium vegetable broth

1 Tbsp chili powder

1 tsp ground cumin

Salt (optional) and pepper to taste

Avocado and lime wedges, for serving

DIRECTIONS:

In a large pot, heat olive oil over medium heat. Add onion and garlic; cook until softened.

Add sweet potatoes, black beans, chipotle peppers, crushed tomatoes, vegetable broth, chili powder, and cumin. Season with salt (if using) and pepper.

Bring to a boil, then reduce heat and simmer for 35-40 minutes, or until the sweet potatoes are tender and the chili has thickened.

Serve hot, topped with avocado slices and a squeeze of lime.

TIPS:

For a smokier flavor, add an extra chipotle pepper.

This chili freezes well for future meals.

N.V.: Calories: 260, Fat: 6g, Carbs: 47g, Protein: 11g, Sugar: 9g

---

3. MOROCCAN-INSPIRED SWEET POTATO AND BLACK BEAN STEW

P.T.: 20 min

C.T.: 40 min

M.C.: Simmering

SERVINGS: 6

INGR.:

2 Tbsp olive oil

1 large onion, finely chopped

2 cloves garlic, minced

2 sweet potatoes, peeled and cubed

1 can (15 oz) black beans, rinsed and drained

1 can (14.5 oz) diced tomatoes, undrained

4 cups low-sodium vegetable broth

1 tsp ground cinnamon

1 tsp ground cumin

1/2 tsp ground turmeric

1/2 cup dried apricots, chopped

Salt (optional) and pepper to taste

Chopped fresh cilantro and toasted almonds, for garnish

DIRECTIONS:

Heat olive oil in a large pot over medium heat. Add onion and garlic; cook until softened.

Add sweet potatoes, black beans, diced tomatoes, vegetable broth, cinnamon, cumin, and turmeric. Season with salt (if using) and pepper.

Bring to a boil, then reduce heat and simmer for 35-40 minutes, until the sweet potatoes are tender.

Stir in dried apricots and simmer for an additional 5 minutes.

Serve hot, garnished with cilantro and toasted almonds.

TIPS:

Serve with couscous for a traditional Moroccan meal.

Add a pinch of cayenne pepper for a spicy kick.

N.V.: Calories: 280, Fat: 5g, Carbs: 55g, Protein: 9g, Sugar: 15g

6.3 BAKED SALMON WITH GARLIC AND DIJON

1. CLASSIC BAKED SALMON WITH GARLIC AND DIJON

P.T.: 10 min

C.T.: 20 min

M.C.: Baking

SERVINGS: 4

INGR.:

4 salmon fillets (6 oz each)

2 Tbsp Dijon mustard

2 cloves garlic, minced

2 Tbsp olive oil

1 Tbsp lemon juice

Salt (optional) and pepper to taste

1 Tbsp fresh dill, chopped

Lemon slices, for garnish

DIRECTIONS:

Preheat oven to 400°F (200°C). Line a baking sheet with parchment paper. In a small bowl, mix together Dijon mustard, garlic, olive oil, lemon juice, salt (if using), and pepper. Place salmon fillets on the prepared baking sheet. Spread the mustard mixture over the top of each fillet. Bake for 18-20 minutes, or until salmon flakes easily with a fork. Garnish with fresh dill and lemon slices before serving.

TIPS:

Ensure the salmon is at room temperature before baking for even cooking. For a crispy top, broil the salmon for the last 2 minutes of cooking.

N.V.: Calories: 290, Fat: 18g, Carbs: 1g, Protein: 30g, Sugar: 0g

P.T.: 15 min

C.T.: 25 min

M.C.: Baking

SERVINGS: 4

INGR.:

4 salmon fillets (6 oz each)

1/4 cup olive oil

2 Tbsp lemon juice

1 Tbsp fresh rosemary, minced

1 Tbsp fresh thyme, minced

2 cloves garlic, minced

Salt (optional) and pepper to taste

Lemon slices and additional herbs, for garnish

DIRECTIONS:

Preheat oven to 375°F (190°C). In a small bowl, combine olive oil, lemon juice, rosemary, thyme, garlic, salt (if using), and pepper.

Place salmon fillets in a baking dish. Pour the herb mixture over the salmon, ensuring each piece is well coated.

Cover with foil and bake for 20 minutes. Uncover and bake for an additional 5 minutes, or until salmon is flaky.

Serve garnished with lemon slices and a sprinkle of fresh herbs.

TIPS:

Marinate the salmon in the herb mixture for up to an hour before baking for deeper flavors.

Pair with a light salad or steamed vegetables for a balanced meal.

N.V.: Calories: 310, Fat: 23g, Carbs: 2g, Protein: 24g, Sugar: 0g

P.T.: 10 min

C.T.: 15 min

M.C.: Baking

SERVINGS: 4

INGR.:

4 salmon fillets (6 oz each)

2 Tbsp Dijon mustard

2 Tbsp honey

1 Tbsp olive oil

1 Tbsp apple cider vinegar

Salt (optional) and pepper to taste

Fresh parsley, chopped for garnish

DIRECTIONS:

Preheat oven to 400°F (200°C). In a bowl, whisk together Dijon mustard, honey, olive oil, apple cider vinegar, salt (if using), and pepper. Place salmon on a greased baking sheet. Brush the glaze over each fillet. Bake for 12-15 minutes, or until the salmon is cooked through and glaze is bubbly. Garnish with chopped parsley before serving.

TIPS:

For an extra kick, add a pinch of red pepper flakes to the glaze. Serve with roasted sweet potatoes or quinoa for a hearty meal.

N.V.: Calories: 295, Fat: 13g, Carbs: 12g, Protein: 31g, Sugar: 11g

4. GARLIC PARMESAN CRUSTED SALMON

P.T.: 15 min

C.T.: 15 min

M.C.: Baking

SERVINGS: 4

INGR.:

4 salmon fillets (6 oz each)

2 Tbsp olive oil

3 cloves garlic, minced

1/2 cup grated Parmesan cheese

1 Tbsp Dijon mustard

1 Tbsp lemon juice

Salt (optional) and pepper to taste

Fresh parsley, for garnish

DIRECTIONS:

Preheat oven to 400°F (200°C). In a bowl, mix olive oil, garlic, Parmesan cheese, Dijon mustard, lemon juice, salt (if using), and pepper.

Place salmon fillets on a greased baking sheet. Spread the Parmesan mixture evenly over each fillet.

Bake for 12-15 minutes, or until the crust is golden and salmon flakes easily with a fork. Garnish with parsley before serving.

TIPS:

Use freshly grated Parmesan for the best flavor and melting quality.

Pair with a Caesar salad for a deliciously themed meal.

N.V.: Calories: 325, Fat: 19g, Carbs: 3g, Protein: 34g, Sugar: 1g

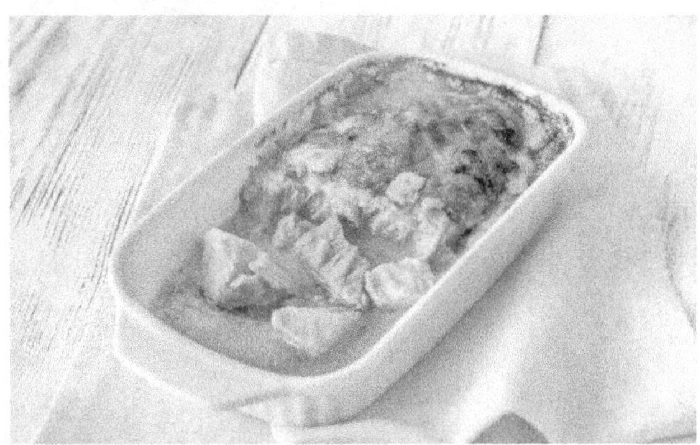

CHAPTER 7: SIDE DISHES TO SAVOR

7.1 ROASTED BRUSSELS SPROUTS WITH ALMONDS

1. ROASTED BRUSSELS SPROUTS WITH ALMONDS AND BALSAMIC GLAZE

P.T.: 10 min

C.T.: 25 min

M.C.: Roasting

SERVINGS: 4

INGR.:

1 lb Brussels sprouts, halved

2 Tbsp olive oil

Salt (optional) and pepper to taste

1/4 cup sliced almonds

2 Tbsp balsamic vinegar

1 Tbsp honey

DIRECTIONS:

Preheat oven to 400°F (200°C). Toss Brussels sprouts with olive oil, salt (if using), and pepper on a baking sheet. Roast for 20 minutes, until tender and caramelized.

In the last 5 minutes of roasting, sprinkle sliced almonds over the Brussels sprouts to toast lightly.

Drizzle balsamic vinegar and honey over the warm Brussels sprouts and almonds; toss to coat evenly.

TIPS:

For added crispiness, broil for the last 2-3 minutes.

Substitute honey with maple syrup for a vegan version.

N.V.: Calories: 180, Fat: 10g, Carbs: 20g, Protein: 6g, Sugar: 9g

2. SAUTÉED BRUSSELS SPROUTS WITH ALMONDS AND GARLIC

P.T.: 10 min

C.T.: 15 min

M.C.: Sautéing

SERVINGS: 4

INGR.:

1 lb Brussels sprouts, trimmed and halved

2 Tbsp olive oil

3 cloves garlic, minced

1/4 cup sliced almonds

Salt (optional) and pepper to taste

Lemon wedges, for serving

DIRECTIONS:

Heat olive oil in a large skillet over medium heat. Add garlic and almonds, sauté until golden. Add Brussels sprouts, season with salt (if using) and pepper. Cook, stirring occasionally, until sprouts are tender and browned, about 12-15 minutes. Serve with lemon wedges on the side.

TIPS:

Keep the heat on medium to prevent garlic from burning.

Squeeze lemon over the Brussels sprouts before serving for a fresh zing.

N.V.: Calories: 160, Fat: 11g, Carbs: 14g, Protein: 5g, Sugar: 3g

3. BRUSSELS SPROUTS WITH CRANBERRIES AND ALMONDS

P.T.: 15 min

C.T.: 20 min

M.C.: Roasting

SERVINGS: 4

INGR.:

1 lb Brussels sprouts, halved

2 Tbsp olive oil

Salt (optional) and pepper to taste

1/3 cup dried cranberries

1/4 cup sliced almonds

2 Tbsp balsamic glaze

DIRECTIONS:

Preheat oven to 375°F (190°C). Toss Brussels sprouts with olive oil, salt (if using), and pepper. Spread on a baking sheet.

Roast for 15 minutes. Add cranberries and almonds; roast for another 5 minutes.

Drizzle with balsamic glaze before serving.

TIPS:

Add a sprinkle of orange zest for a citrus note.

Perfect as a holiday side dish or to add color and texture to any meal.

N.V.: Calories: 190, Fat: 9g, Carbs: 25g, Protein: 5g, Sugar: 13g

4. CREAMY BRUSSELS SPROUTS WITH ALMONDS

P.T.: 10 min

C.T.: 15 min

M.C.: Sautéing

SERVINGS: 4

INGR.:

1 lb Brussels sprouts, halved

1 Tbsp olive oil

1/4 cup sliced almonds

1/2 cup low-fat milk

1 Tbsp flour

Salt (optional) and pepper to taste

Nutmeg, a pinch

DIRECTIONS:

In a large skillet, heat olive oil over medium heat. Add Brussels sprouts and cook until they start to brown, about 8-10 minutes.

Stir in almonds, cooking until toasted, about 2 minutes.

Sprinkle flour over the sprouts and almonds; stir to coat. Slowly add milk, stirring constantly, until the mixture thickens. Season with salt (if using), pepper, and nutmeg.

Serve warm as a creamy side dish.

TIPS:

Use almond milk for a dairy-free version.

Great alongside roasted meats or as a vegetarian main with quinoa.

N.V.: Calories: 160, Fat: 8g, Carbs: 18g, Protein: 6g, Sugar: 5g

7.2 CAULIFLOWER MASH

1. CLASSIC GARLIC CAULIFLOWER MASH

P.T.: 10 min

C.T.: 20 min

M.C.: Boiling/Blending

SERVINGS: 4

INGR.:

1 large head of cauliflower, cut into florets

4 cloves garlic, peeled

2 Tbsp olive oil

1/4 cup grated Parmesan cheese

Salt (optional) and pepper to taste

1/4 cup unsweetened almond milk

DIRECTIONS:

In a large pot, bring water to a boil. Add cauliflower florets and garlic cloves; cook until cauliflower is very tender, about 15 minutes.

Drain cauliflower and garlic; transfer to a food processor. Add olive oil, Parmesan cheese, salt (if using), pepper, and almond milk.

Blend until smooth and creamy. Adjust seasoning as needed.

TIPS:

For a richer flavor, roast the garlic before adding it to the mash.

Serve with a drizzle of olive oil and a sprinkle of fresh herbs for garnish.

N.V.: Calories: 150, Fat: 10g, Carbs: 10g, Protein: 5g, Sugar: 4g

2. ROASTED CAULIFLOWER AND GARLIC MASH WITH CHIVES

P.T.: 15 min

C.T.: 25 min

M.C.: Roasting/Blending

SERVINGS: 4

INGR.:

1 head of cauliflower, cut into florets

6 cloves garlic, unpeeled

3 Tbsp olive oil, divided

Salt (optional) and pepper to taste

2 Tbsp chopped chives

1/4 cup unsweetened almond milk

DIRECTIONS:

Preheat oven to 425°F (220°C). Toss cauliflower and garlic cloves with 2 tablespoons of olive oil and season with salt (if using) and pepper. Roast for 25 minutes, until tender and golden.

Squeeze the roasted garlic out of its skin and place in a food processor with the cauliflower. Add remaining olive oil, almond milk, and chives. Blend until smooth.

Serve garnished with additional chives.

TIPS:

Roasting the cauliflower adds depth to the mash's flavor.

Great as a side dish for grilled or roasted meats.

N.V.: Calories: 160, Fat: 11g, Carbs: 13g, Protein: 5g, Sugar: 5g

P.T.: 10 min

C.T.: 20 min

M.C.: Steaming/Blending

SERVINGS: 4

INGR.:

1 large head of cauliflower, cut into florets

1/4 cup fresh parsley, chopped

1/4 cup fresh basil, chopped

2 Tbsp olive oil

Salt (optional) and pepper to taste

1/4 cup unsweetened almond milk

1 Tbsp lemon zest

DIRECTIONS:

Steam cauliflower until very tender, about 15-20 minutes.

Transfer steamed cauliflower to a food processor. Add parsley, basil, olive oil, salt (if using), pepper, almond milk, and lemon zest. Blend until smooth and creamy. Adjust seasoning as needed.

TIPS:

The lemon zest adds a bright, refreshing note to the mash.

Perfect alongside fish or poultry for a light, healthful meal.

N.V.: Calories: 120, Fat: 7g, Carbs: 12g, Protein: 4g, Sugar: 5g

P.T.: 10 min

C.T.: 20 min

M.C.: Boiling/Blending

SERVINGS: 4

INGR.:

1 large head cauliflower, cut into florets

1/2 cup shredded sharp cheddar cheese

2 Tbsp unsalted butter

1/4 cup Greek yogurt

Salt (optional) and pepper to taste

1/4 tsp garlic powder

DIRECTIONS:

Bring a large pot of water to a boil. Add cauliflower florets and cook until very tender, about 15 minutes. Drain well.

Transfer the cauliflower to a food processor. Add cheddar cheese, butter, Greek yogurt, salt (if using), pepper, and garlic powder. Blend until smooth and creamy. Adjust the seasoning as necessary.

TIPS:

For a smoother texture, process the cauliflower in batches.

Garnish with extra shredded cheese and a sprinkle of paprika before serving for added flavor and color.

N.V.: Calories: 190, Fat: 14g, Carbs: 9g, Protein: 9g, Sugar: 4g

5. SPICY CAULIFLOWER MASH WITH JALAPEÑOS

P.T.: 10 min

C.T.: 20 min

M.C.: Steaming/Blending

SERVINGS: 4

INGR.:

1 head of cauliflower, cut into florets

1 Tbsp olive oil

2 Tbsp pickled jalapeños, chopped

1/4 cup unsweetened almond milk

Salt (optional) and pepper to taste

1/4 tsp cumin

Fresh cilantro, for garnish

DIRECTIONS:

Steam the cauliflower florets until tender, about 15-20 minutes.

Transfer the cauliflower to a food processor. Add olive oil, pickled jalapeños, almond milk, salt (if using), pepper, and cumin.

Blend until smooth. Adjust seasoning as needed.

Garnish with fresh cilantro before serving.

TIPS:

For a milder mash, reduce the amount of jalapeños.

Serve as a side to grilled meats for a meal with a kick.

N.V.: Calories: 80, Fat: 4g, Carbs: 10g, Protein: 3g, Sugar: 4g

6. MEDITERRANEAN CAULIFLOWER MASH

P.T.: 15 min

C.T.: 20 min

M.C.: Boiling/Blending

SERVINGS: 4

INGR.:

1 large head cauliflower, cut into florets

2 Tbsp olive oil

1/4 cup sun-dried tomatoes, chopped

1/4 cup kalamata olives, pitted and chopped

2 Tbsp capers, rinsed

Salt (optional) and pepper to taste

1 Tbsp fresh lemon juice

1/4 tsp dried oregano

DIRECTIONS:

In a large pot, boil cauliflower florets until tender, about 15 minutes. Drain well.

In a food processor, combine boiled cauliflower, olive oil, sun-dried tomatoes, kalamata olives, capers, salt (if using), pepper, lemon juice, and oregano.

Blend until smooth. Adjust seasoning as necessary.

Serve garnished with additional chopped olives and sun-dried tomatoes if desired.

TIPS:

Adding a sprinkle of feta cheese on top before serving introduces an extra layer of Mediterranean flavor.

This mash pairs wonderfully with fish or poultry for a complete and flavorful meal.

N.V.: Calories: 150, Fat: 10g, Carbs: 13g, Protein: 4g, Sugar: 6g

7.3 QUINOA AND BLACK BEAN SALAD

1. CLASSIC QUINOA AND BLACK BEAN SALAD

P.T.: 15 min

C.T.: 20 min

M.C.: Boiling/Mixing

SERVINGS: 4

INGR.:

1 cup quinoa, rinsed

1 can (15 oz) black beans, drained and rinsed

1 red bell pepper, diced

1/4 cup fresh cilantro, chopped

1/4 cup lime juice

2 Tbsp olive oil

Salt (optional) and pepper to taste

1 avocado, diced

1/4 cup red onion, finely chopped

DIRECTIONS:

In a medium saucepan, bring 2 cups of water to a boil. Add quinoa, reduce heat to low, cover, and simmer until quinoa is tender and water is absorbed, about 15 minutes. Let cool.

In a large bowl, combine cooled quinoa, black beans, red bell pepper, cilantro, lime juice, olive oil, salt (if using), pepper, avocado, and red onion.

Toss gently to combine. Serve chilled or at room temperature.

TIPS:

To enhance the flavor, let the salad chill for an hour before serving.

Add grilled corn or cherry tomatoes for extra freshness and color.

N.V.: Calories: 320, Fat: 14g, Carbs: 42g, Protein: 10g, Sugar: 3g

2. MEDITERRANEAN QUINOA AND BLACK BEAN SALAD

P.T.: 15 min

C.T.: 20 min

M.C.: Boiling/Mixing

SERVINGS: 4

INGR.:

1 cup quinoa, rinsed

1 can (15 oz) black beans, drained and rinsed

1 cucumber, diced

1/2 cup Kalamata olives, pitted and halved

1/2 cup feta cheese, crumbled

1/4 cup sun-dried tomatoes, chopped

1/4 cup olive oil

3 Tbsp lemon juice

1 tsp dried oregano

Salt (optional) and pepper to taste

DIRECTIONS:

Cook quinoa as directed in recipe 1. Let cool.

In a large bowl, combine quinoa, black beans, cucumber, Kalamata olives, feta cheese, sun-dried tomatoes, olive oil, lemon juice, oregano, salt (if using), and pepper.

Toss until well combined. Serve chilled or at room temperature.

TIPS:

For added texture, include a handful of pine nuts or slivered almonds.

Perfect as a side dish or a light main course.

N.V.: Calories: 350, Fat: 18g, Carbs: 40g, Protein: 12g, Sugar: 4g

<hr>

3. SPICY SOUTHWEST QUINOA AND BLACK BEAN SALAD

P.T.: 15 min

C.T.: 20 min

M.C.: Boiling/Mixing

SERVINGS: 4

INGR.:

1 cup quinoa, rinsed

1 can (15 oz) black beans, drained and rinsed

1 cup corn kernels, fresh or frozen (thawed)

1 red bell pepper, diced

1/4 cup fresh cilantro, chopped

2 Tbsp lime juice

1 Tbsp olive oil

1/2 tsp cumin

1/4 tsp chili powder

Salt (optional) and pepper to taste

1 avocado, diced

1/4 cup red onion, finely chopped

DIRECTIONS:

Cook quinoa as instructed in recipe 1. Let cool.

In a large bowl, mix quinoa, black beans, corn, red bell pepper, cilantro, lime juice, olive oil, cumin, chili powder, salt (if using), pepper, avocado, and red onion.

Toss to combine. Serve chilled or at room temperature.

TIPS:

Add a diced jalapeño for extra heat.

Serve with tortilla chips for a crunchy texture.

N.V.: Calories: 330, Fat: 15g, Carbs: 45g, Protein: 11g, Sugar: 5g

<hr>

4. TROPICAL QUINOA AND BLACK BEAN SALAD

P.T.: 15 min

C.T.: 20 min

M.C.: Boiling/Mixing

SERVINGS: 4

INGR.:

1 cup quinoa, rinsed

1 can (15 oz) black beans, drained and rinsed

1 mango, diced

1/2 cup pineapple, diced

1 red bell pepper, diced

1/4 cup fresh cilantro, chopped

2 Tbsp lime juice

1 Tbsp olive oil

Salt (optional) and pepper to taste

1/4 cup coconut flakes, toasted

DIRECTIONS:

Cook quinoa according to package instructions and let cool.

In a large bowl, combine cooled quinoa, black beans, mango, pineapple, red bell pepper, cilantro, lime juice, olive oil, salt (if using), and pepper.

Toss until everything is well mixed. Garnish with toasted coconut flakes before serving.

TIPS:

For an extra protein boost, add grilled shrimp or chicken.

Ensure the mango and pineapple are ripe for the best flavor.

N.V.: Calories: 310, Fat: 9g, Carbs: 52g, Protein: 9g, Sugar: 15g

5. QUINOA AND BLACK BEAN SALAD WITH AVOCADO LIME DRESSING

P.T.: 20 min

C.T.: 20 min

M.C.: Boiling/Blending

SERVINGS: 4

INGR.:

1 cup quinoa, rinsed

1 can (15 oz) black beans, drained and rinsed

1 cup cherry tomatoes, halved

1 cucumber, diced

1/4 cup red onion, finely chopped

For the dressing:

1 ripe avocado

2 Tbsp lime juice

1/4 cup cilantro leaves

2 Tbsp olive oil

Salt (optional) and pepper to taste

Water, as needed for consistency

DIRECTIONS:

Cook quinoa according to package instructions and let cool.

For the dressing, blend avocado, lime juice, cilantro, olive oil, salt (if using), and pepper until smooth. Add water as needed to achieve desired consistency.

In a large bowl, combine cooled quinoa, black beans, cherry tomatoes, cucumber, and red onion.

Pour the dressing over the salad and toss until well coated. Serve chilled or at room temperature.

TIPS:

The dressing can be made ahead and stored in the fridge for up to 2 days.

Add crumbled feta or goat cheese for a creamy texture and extra flavor.

N.V.: Calories: 350, Fat: 15g, Carbs: 45g, Protein: 11g, Sugar: 6g

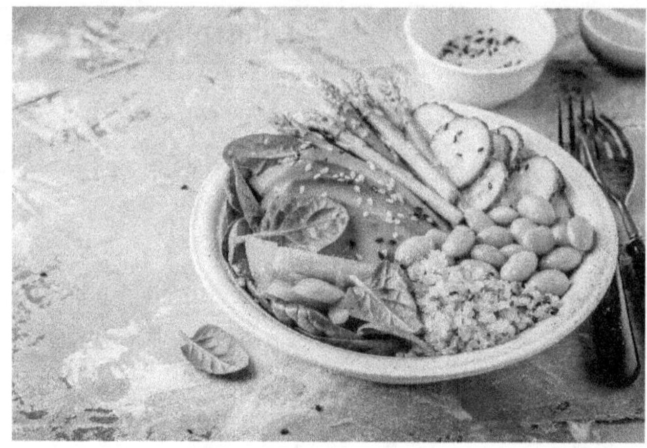

CHAPTER 8: DASH-FRIENDLY DESSERT

8.1 BERRY AND CHIA SEED PUDDING

1. CLASSIC BERRY AND CHIA SEED PUDDING

P.T.: 10 min

C.T.: 0 min (plus refrigeration time)

M.C.: Refrigeration

SERVINGS: 4

INGR.:

½ cup chia seeds

2 cups almond milk

1 Tbsp honey or maple syrup

1 tsp vanilla extract

1 cup mixed berries (strawberries, blueberries, raspberries)

PROCEDURE:

In a bowl, whisk together chia seeds, almond milk, honey (or maple syrup), and vanilla extract until well combined.

Let the mixture sit for 5 minutes, then whisk again to prevent clumping.

Cover and refrigerate for at least 2 hours, or overnight, until the mixture achieves a pudding-like consistency.

Serve the pudding topped with mixed berries.

TIPS:

For the best texture, let the pudding set overnight in the refrigerator.

Add a layer of berry compote at the bottom of the serving dish for an extra burst of flavor.

N.V.: Calories: 200, Fat: 9g, Carbs: 24g, Protein: 5g, Sugar: 10g

2. LEMON RASPBERRY CHIA SEED PUDDING

P.T.: 10 min

C.T.: 0 min (plus refrigeration time)

M.C.: Refrigeration

SERVINGS: 4

INGR.:

½ cup chia seeds

2 cups coconut milk

1 Tbsp honey or maple syrup

1 lemon, zested and juiced

1 cup fresh raspberries

PROCEDURE:

Combine chia seeds, coconut milk, honey (or maple syrup), lemon zest, and lemon juice in

a mixing bowl. Stir well to integrate all the ingredients and let sit for 5 minutes, then stir again to break up any clumps.

Refrigerate for 2 hours or overnight until set.

Top with fresh raspberries before serving.

TIPS:

Mixing the lemon zest into the pudding adds a refreshing citrus flavor that complements the raspberries.

For a smoother texture, blend the raspberries into the milk before adding the chia seeds.

N.V.: Calories: 210, Fat: 12g, Carbs: 23g, Protein: 5g, Sugar: 11g

P.T.: 10 min

C.T.: 0 min (plus refrigeration time)

M.C.: Refrigeration

SERVINGS: 4

INGR.:

½ cup chia seeds

2 cups almond milk

1 Tbsp honey or maple syrup

½ tsp almond extract

1 cup blueberries

¼ cup sliced almonds, toasted

PROCEDURE:

In a bowl, combine chia seeds, almond milk, honey (or maple syrup), and almond extract, stirring well to mix.

Let the mixture sit for a few minutes, then stir again to ensure there are no clumps.

Refrigerate the mixture for at least 2 hours, preferably overnight, until it thickens into a pudding consistency.

Serve the pudding topped with fresh blueberries and sprinkled with toasted sliced almonds.

TIPS:

Toasting the almonds before adding them to the pudding will enhance their flavor and add a pleasant crunch.

For a layered dessert, alternate layers of chia pudding and mashed blueberries in serving glasses.

N.V.: Calories: 220, Fat: 11g, Carbs: 26g, Protein: 6g, Sugar: 12g

P.T.: 10 min

C.T.: 0 min (plus refrigeration time)

M.C.: Refrigeration

SERVINGS: 4

INGR.:

½ cup chia seeds

2 cups cashew milk

1 Tbsp honey or maple syrup

1 tsp vanilla extract

1 cup strawberries, sliced

1 kiwi, peeled and sliced

PROCEDURE:

Mix chia seeds, cashew milk, honey (or maple syrup), and vanilla extract in a bowl until well combined. Let the mixture rest for a few minutes, then stir again to prevent clumping.

Refrigerate for a minimum of 2 hours, or overnight, until it reaches a pudding consistency. Top with sliced strawberries and kiwi before serving.

TIPS:

For a more vibrant flavor, macerate the strawberries in a teaspoon of sugar or honey before adding them to the pudding. Layer the pudding with slices of strawberries and kiwi in clear glasses for an appealing presentation.

N.V.: Calories: 210, Fat: 8g, Carbs: 30g, Protein: 5g, Sugar: 13g

8.2 GRILLED PEACHES WITH CINNAMON

1. CLASSIC GRILLED PEACHES WITH CINNAMON HONEY DRIZZLE

P.T.: 10 min

C.T.: 10 min

M.C.: Grilling

SERVINGS: 4

INGR.:

4 ripe peaches, halved and pitted

1 Tbsp olive oil

2 tsp cinnamon

4 Tbsp honey

PROCEDURE:

Preheat the grill to medium-high heat.

Brush the cut sides of the peaches with olive oil and sprinkle with cinnamon.

Place peaches cut-side down on the grill and cook for about 5 minutes, or until grill marks appear.

Flip the peaches and grill for another 5 minutes until tender.

Drizzle honey over the grilled peaches and serve warm.

TIPS:

Choose peaches that are ripe but still firm to hold up well on the grill.

For an extra flavor dimension, add a pinch of nutmeg or clove along with the cinnamon.

N.V.: Calories: 150, Fat: 3.5g, Carbs: 31g, Protein: 1g, Sugar: 28g

2. GRILLED PEACHES WITH CINNAMON AND VANILLA YOGURT

P.T.: 10 min

C.T.: 10 min

M.C.: Grilling

SERVINGS: 4

INGR.:

4 ripe peaches, halved and pitted

1 Tbsp olive oil

2 tsp cinnamon

1 cup low-fat vanilla yogurt

PROCEDURE:

Preheat the grill to medium-high heat.

Brush the peaches with olive oil and sprinkle with cinnamon.

Grill peaches cut-side down for 5 minutes until they have grill marks.

Flip and continue grilling until they are soft, about another 5 minutes.

Serve the grilled peaches with a dollop of vanilla yogurt on top.

TIPS:

The vanilla yogurt can be mixed with a little honey or maple syrup for added sweetness if desired.

Garnish with fresh mint leaves for a refreshing touch.

N.V.: Calories: 120, Fat: 3g, Carbs: 22g, Protein: 3g, Sugar: 20g

P.T.: 15 min

C.T.: 20 min

M.C.: Grilling and simmering

SERVINGS: 4

INGR.:

4 ripe peaches, halved and pitted

2 tsp olive oil

1 tsp ground cinnamon

½ cup balsamic vinegar

2 Tbsp brown sugar

PROCEDURE:

Preheat the grill to medium-high heat.

Brush peaches with olive oil and sprinkle with cinnamon.

Grill peaches cut-side down for about 5 minutes until grill marks form, then turn over and grill for another 5 minutes.

In a small saucepan, combine balsamic vinegar and brown sugar. Simmer over medium heat until the mixture reduces by half and thickens into a syrup, about 10 minutes.

Drizzle the balsamic reduction over the grilled peaches and serve warm.

TIPS:

The balsamic reduction can be made in advance and stored in the refrigerator.

Serve with a sprinkle of crushed walnuts or pecans for added texture.

N.V.: Calories: 160, Fat: 3g, Carbs: 33g, Protein: 1g, Sugar: 30g

P.T.: 15 min

C.T.: 10 min

M.C.: Grilling

SERVINGS: 4

INGR.:

4 ripe peaches, halved and pitted

2 tsp olive oil

1 tsp cinnamon

1 cup ricotta cheese

2 Tbsp honey

½ tsp vanilla extract

PROCEDURE:

Preheat the grill to medium-high heat.

Brush peaches with olive oil and sprinkle with cinnamon. Grill peaches cut-side down for about 5 minutes, then flip and grill for another 5 minutes until tender.

In a small bowl, mix ricotta cheese, honey, and vanilla extract until smooth.

Serve grilled peaches topped with a dollop of ricotta cream.

TIPS:

For added sweetness and flavor, mix a little orange zest into the ricotta cream.

If the ricotta mixture is too thick, thin it with a little milk or cream to desired consistency.

N.V.: Calories: 200, Fat: 8g, Carbs: 28g, Protein: 7g, Sugar: 24g

8.3 WHOLE WHEAT BANANA BREAD

1. CLASSIC WHOLE WHEAT BANANA BREAD

P.T.: 15 min

C.T.: 55 min

M.C.: Baking

SERVINGS: 10 slices

INGR.:

1¾ cups whole wheat flour

1 tsp baking soda

½ tsp salt

⅓ cup olive oil or melted coconut oil

½ cup honey or maple syrup

2 large eggs

1 cup mashed ripe bananas (about 2-3 bananas)

¼ cup water

1 tsp vanilla extract

½ cup walnuts, chopped (optional)

PROCEDURE:

Preheat the oven to 325°F (165°C). Grease a 9x5-inch loaf pan.

In a large bowl, whisk together whole wheat flour, baking soda, and salt.

In another bowl, mix olive oil, honey, eggs, mashed bananas, water, and vanilla extract.

Add the wet ingredients to the dry ingredients, mixing until just combined. Fold in walnuts if using.

Pour the batter into the prepared loaf pan and smooth the top.

Bake for 55-60 minutes or until a toothpick inserted into the center comes out clean.

Let the bread cool in the pan for 10 minutes, then turn out onto a wire rack to cool completely.

TIPS:

Ensure the bananas are very ripe for the best sweetness and moisture.

Add a tablespoon of ground flaxseed or chia seeds to the batter for an extra boost of omega-3 fatty acids.

N.V.: Calories: 230, Fat: 9g, Carbs: 35g, Protein: 4g, Sugar: 16g

2. WHOLE WHEAT BANANA BREAD WITH BLUEBERRIES

P.T.: 15 min

C.T.: 55 min

M.C.: Baking

SERVINGS: 10 slices

INGR.:

1¾ cups whole wheat flour

1 tsp baking soda

½ tsp salt

⅓ cup olive oil or melted coconut oil

½ cup honey or maple syrup

2 large eggs

1 cup mashed ripe bananas

¼ cup milk or almond milk

1 tsp vanilla extract

1 cup fresh or frozen blueberries

PROCEDURE:

Preheat the oven to 325°F (165°C). Grease a 9x5-inch loaf pan.

In a large bowl, combine whole wheat flour, baking soda, and salt.

In a separate bowl, whisk together olive oil, honey, eggs, mashed bananas, milk, and vanilla extract.

Gently fold the wet ingredients into the dry ingredients until just combined, being careful not to overmix.

Carefully fold in the blueberries.

Pour the batter into the prepared loaf pan and smooth the top.

Bake for 55-60 minutes, or until a toothpick inserted into the center comes out clean.

Cool in the pan for 10 minutes, then transfer to a wire rack to cool completely.

TIPS:

If using frozen blueberries, do not thaw them before adding to the batter to prevent discoloration.

Lemon zest can be added to the batter for a refreshing citrus flavor that complements the blueberries.

N.V.: Calories: 240, Fat: 9g, Carbs: 37g, Protein: 4g, Sugar: 17g

---

3. WHOLE WHEAT BANANA BREAD WITH CINNAMON SWIRL

P.T.: 20 min

C.T.: 60 min

M.C.: Baking

SERVINGS: 10 slices

INGR.:

1¾ cups whole wheat flour

1 tsp baking soda

½ tsp salt

⅓ cup unsalted butter, melted

½ cup honey or maple syrup

2 large eggs

1 cup mashed ripe bananas

¼ cup milk

1 tsp vanilla extract

For the Cinnamon Swirl:

1 Tbsp ground cinnamon

3 Tbsp brown sugar

PROCEDURE:

Preheat oven to 325°F (165°C). Grease and flour a 9x5-inch loaf pan.

Mix whole wheat flour, baking soda, and salt in a bowl.

In another bowl, combine melted butter, honey, eggs, mashed bananas, milk, and vanilla extract.

Gradually mix the wet ingredients into the dry ingredients, stirring until just combined.

Mix cinnamon and brown sugar in a small bowl.

Pour half of the banana bread batter into the loaf pan. Sprinkle half of the cinnamon sugar mixture over the batter.

Add the remaining batter, then top with the rest of the cinnamon sugar mixture. Use a knife to swirl the cinnamon sugar into the batter.

Bake for 60 minutes, or until a toothpick inserted into the center comes out clean.

Cool in the pan for 10 minutes, then remove to a wire rack to cool completely.

TIPS:

For a more pronounced swirl, layer the cinnamon sugar between layers of batter more evenly.

The bread's flavor enhances if left to sit for a day, allowing the cinnamon and banana flavors to meld.

N.V.: Calories: 250, Fat: 8g, Carbs: 42g, Protein: 5g, Sugar: 20g

4. CHOCOLATE CHIP WHOLE WHEAT BANANA BREAD

P.T.: 15 min

C.T.: 55 min

M.C.: Baking

SERVINGS: 10 slices

INGR.:

1¾ cups whole wheat flour

1 tsp baking soda

½ tsp salt

⅓ cup vegetable oil

½ cup honey or maple syrup

2 large eggs

1 cup mashed ripe bananas

¼ cup water

1 tsp vanilla extract

½ cup dark chocolate chips

PROCEDURE:

Preheat the oven to 325°F (165°C). Grease a 9x5-inch loaf pan.

Combine whole wheat flour, baking soda, and salt in a bowl.

In a separate bowl, mix vegetable oil, honey, eggs, mashed bananas, water, and vanilla extract. Gradually add the wet ingredients to the dry, stirring until just combined. Fold in the chocolate chips. Pour the batter into the prepared loaf pan, smoothing the top with a spatula. Bake for 55-60 minutes or until a toothpick inserted into the center comes out clean. Allow cooling in the pan for 10 minutes, then transfer to a wire rack to cool completely.

TIPS:

For a healthier version, opt for dark chocolate chips with a higher cocoa content. Adding a pinch of espresso powder can enhance the chocolate flavor without adding noticeable coffee taste.

N.V.: Calories: 270, Fat: 10g, Carbs: 42g, Protein: 5g, Sugar: 22g

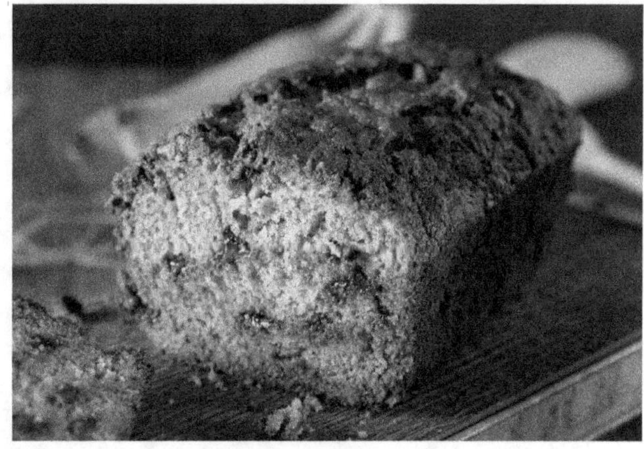

CHAPTER 9: HEARTY SOUPS AND STEWS

9.1 LENTIL AND SPINACH SOUP

1. CLASSIC LENTIL AND SPINACH SOUP

P.T.: 10 min

C.T.: 45 min

M.C.: Simmering

SERVINGS: 4

INGR.:

1 cup dried green lentils, rinsed

1 Tbsp olive oil

1 onion, chopped

2 garlic cloves, minced

2 carrots, diced

4 cups vegetable broth

2 cups water

1 tsp ground cumin

½ tsp ground coriander

Salt and pepper to taste

2 cups fresh spinach, chopped

PROCEDURE:

Heat olive oil in a large pot over medium heat. Add onion, garlic, and carrots, sautéing until softened.

Stir in lentils, vegetable broth, water, cumin, and coriander. Bring to a boil, then reduce heat and simmer, covered, for 30 minutes or until lentils are tender.

Add spinach and cook until wilted, about 5 minutes. Season with salt and pepper.

Serve hot, adjusting seasoning as needed.

TIPS:

For a creamier texture, blend part of the soup and then mix it back in.

Add a squeeze of lemon juice before serving to enhance the flavors.

N.V.: Calories: 220, Fat: 4g, Carbs: 35g, Protein: 14g, Sugar: 5g

2. MEDITERRANEAN LENTIL AND SPINACH SOUP

P.T.: 15 min

C.T.: 40 min

M.C.: Simmering

SERVINGS: 4

INGR.:

1 cup red lentils, rinsed

1 Tbsp olive oil

1 onion, finely chopped

3 garlic cloves, minced

1 red bell pepper, diced

4 cups vegetable broth

1 can (14 oz) diced tomatoes

1 tsp dried oregano

1 tsp dried basil

Salt and pepper to taste

2 cups fresh spinach, chopped

Fresh parsley, chopped (for garnish)

PROCEDURE:

In a large pot, heat olive oil over medium heat. Sauté onion, garlic, and red bell pepper until softened.

Add red lentils, vegetable broth, diced tomatoes, oregano, and basil. Season with salt and pepper.

Bring to a boil, then reduce heat and simmer, partially covered, for 25-30 minutes, until lentils are fully cooked.

Stir in spinach and cook until wilted, about 3 minutes.

Garnish with fresh parsley and serve warm.

TIPS:

Serve with a side of whole-grain bread or a slice of rustic sourdough for a complete meal.

A splash of balsamic vinegar can add a nice depth of flavor to the soup.

N.V.: Calories: 230, Fat: 5g, Carbs: 37g, Protein: 15g, Sugar: 6g

---

3. COCONUT CURRY LENTIL AND SPINACH SOUP

P.T.: 15 min

C.T.: 30 min

M.C.: Simmering

SERVINGS: 4

INGR.:

1 cup yellow lentils, rinsed

1 Tbsp coconut oil

1 onion, chopped

2 garlic cloves, minced

1 Tbsp curry powder

½ tsp ground turmeric

1 can (14 oz) coconut milk

4 cups vegetable broth

Salt and pepper to taste

2 cups fresh spinach, chopped

Fresh cilantro, chopped (for garnish)

PROCEDURE:

In a large pot, heat coconut oil over medium heat. Sauté onion and garlic until translucent.

Stir in curry powder, turmeric, and yellow lentils until well coated with the spices.

Pour in coconut milk and vegetable broth, season with salt and pepper, and bring to a boil.

Reduce heat and simmer for about 20 minutes, or until lentils are tender.

Add spinach, cooking just until wilted, about 3 minutes.

Garnish with fresh cilantro and serve hot.

TIPS:

Adjust the amount of curry powder to control the spice level according to your preference.

Serve with a side of naan or basmati rice for a heartier meal.

N.V.: Calories: 350, Fat: 18g, Carbs: 36g, Protein: 15g, Sugar: 4g

---

4. ITALIAN LENTIL AND SPINACH SOUP WITH TOMATOES

P.T.: 15 min

C.T.: 40 min

M.C.: Simmering

SERVINGS: 4

INGR.:

1 cup brown lentils, rinsed

1 Tbsp olive oil

1 small onion, diced

2 garlic cloves, minced

1 carrot, diced

1 stalk celery, diced

4 cups vegetable broth

1 can (14 oz) crushed tomatoes

1 tsp dried Italian herbs

Salt and pepper to taste

2 cups fresh spinach, chopped

Parmesan cheese, grated (optional, for serving)

PROCEDURE:

Heat olive oil in a large pot over medium heat. Sauté onion, garlic, carrot, and celery until soft.

Add lentils, vegetable broth, crushed tomatoes, and Italian herbs. Season with salt and pepper.

Bring to a boil, then reduce heat and simmer, covered, for about 30 minutes or until lentils are tender.

Stir in spinach and cook until wilted, about 5 minutes.

Serve hot, topped with grated Parmesan cheese if desired.

TIPS:

A splash of red wine added with the broth can enhance the richness of the soup.

For a vegan option, omit the Parmesan or use a plant-based cheese alternative.

N.V.: Calories: 280, Fat: 5g, Carbs: 45g, Protein: 17g, Sugar: 9g

9.2 CHICKEN TORTILLA SOUP

1. CLASSIC CHICKEN TORTILLA SOUP

P.T.: 20 min

C.T.: 30 min

M.C.: Simmering

SERVINGS: 4

INGR.:

2 chicken breasts, cooked and shredded

1 Tbsp olive oil

1 onion, chopped

2 garlic cloves, minced

1 jalapeño, seeded and diced

1 tsp ground cumin

1 tsp chili powder

4 cups chicken broth

1 can (14 oz) diced tomatoes, with juice

1 cup frozen corn kernels

Salt and pepper to taste

4 corn tortillas, cut into strips

Fresh cilantro, chopped (for garnish)

Lime wedges (for serving)

PROCEDURE:

In a large pot, heat olive oil over medium heat. Sauté onion, garlic, and jalapeño until soft.

Stir in cumin, chili powder, chicken broth, diced tomatoes, and corn. Bring to a simmer.

Add the shredded chicken to the pot and

season with salt and pepper. Simmer for 20 minutes.

Meanwhile, bake tortilla strips in the oven at 375°F (190°C) until crispy, about 10-15 minutes.

Serve the soup in bowls, topped with crispy tortilla strips, fresh cilantro, and a squeeze of lime juice.

TIPS:

For a smoky flavor, add a chipotle pepper in adobo sauce to the soup while simmering.

The soup can be thickened with mashed beans or corn tortillas dissolved into the broth.

N.V.: Calories: 250, Fat: 6g, Carbs: 27g, Protein: 25g, Sugar: 5g

2. CREAMY CHICKEN TORTILLA SOUP

P.T.: 20 min

C.T.: 30 min

M.C.: Simmering

SERVINGS: 4

INGR.:

2 chicken breasts, cooked and shredded

1 Tbsp olive oil

1 onion, chopped

2 garlic cloves, minced

1 tsp ground cumin

1 tsp smoked paprika

4 cups chicken broth

1 cup corn kernels

1 can (14 oz) black beans, rinsed and drained

½ cup heavy cream or coconut milk

Salt and pepper to taste

Tortilla strips, for garnish

Avocado slices, for garnish

PROCEDURE:

In a large pot, heat the olive oil over medium heat. Sauté the onion and garlic until translucent.

Add cumin, smoked paprika, chicken broth, corn, and black beans. Bring to a simmer.

Stir in the shredded chicken and heavy cream (or coconut milk). Season with salt and pepper. Cook for another 10 minutes until heated through.

Serve the soup garnished with tortilla strips and avocado slices.

TIPS:

Add a squeeze of lime juice to the soup before serving to brighten the flavors.

For a dairy-free version, use coconut milk to add creaminess without lactose.

N.V.: Calories: 300, Fat: 12g, Carbs: 28g, Protein: 25g, Sugar: 4g

3. SPICY CHICKEN TORTILLA SOUP

P.T.: 20 min

C.T.: 30 min

M.C.: Simmering

SERVINGS: 4

INGR.:

2 chicken breasts, cooked and shredded

1 Tbsp vegetable oil

1 onion, diced

3 garlic cloves, minced

2 jalapeños, diced (leave seeds for extra heat)

1 tsp ground cumin

1 tsp chili powder

4 cups low-sodium chicken broth

1 can (14 oz) fire-roasted diced tomatoes

1 can (14 oz) black beans, rinsed and drained

1 cup frozen corn

Salt and pepper to taste

Tortilla strips, for garnish

Diced avocado and fresh cilantro, for serving

PROCEDURE:

In a large pot, heat oil over medium heat. Add onion, garlic, and jalapeños, sautéing until onion is translucent.

Stir in cumin and chili powder, cooking for 1 minute.

Add chicken broth, diced tomatoes, black beans, and corn. Season with salt and pepper. Bring to a boil, then simmer for 20 minutes.

Add shredded chicken and heat through.

Serve hot, topped with tortilla strips, avocado, and cilantro.

TIPS:

For deeper flavor, add a teaspoon of smoked paprika.

Serve with lime wedges on the side to adjust acidity to taste.

N.V.: Calories: 290, Fat: 8g, Carbs: 33g, Protein: 27g, Sugar: 6g

---

4. VEGETARIAN CHICKEN TORTILLA SOUP (USING PLANT-BASED CHICKEN)

P.T.: 15 min

C.T.: 30 min

M.C.: Simmering

SERVINGS: 4

INGR.:

2 cups plant-based chicken strips

1 Tbsp olive oil

1 large onion, chopped

2 garlic cloves, minced

1 red bell pepper, diced

1 tsp ground cumin

1 tsp paprika

4 cups vegetable broth

1 can (14 oz) diced tomatoes

1 can (14 oz) black beans, rinsed and drained

1 cup corn kernels

Salt and pepper to taste

Tortilla strips and lime wedges, for serving

PROCEDURE:

In a large pot, heat olive oil over medium heat. Sauté onion, garlic, and bell pepper until soft.

Stir in cumin and paprika, cook for 1 minute.

Add vegetable broth, diced tomatoes, black beans, and corn. Season with salt and pepper, and bring to a simmer.

Add plant-based chicken strips and simmer for about 15 minutes.

Adjust seasoning as needed and serve with tortilla strips and lime wedges.

TIPS:

Enhance the soup with a dash of chipotle chili powder for a smoky taste.

Garnish with diced avocado or vegan cheese for extra creaminess.

N.V.: Calories: 270, Fat: 6g, Carbs: 40g, Protein: 20g, Sugar: 7g

<hr>

5. SLOW COOKER CHICKEN TORTILLA SOUP

P.T.: 15 min

C.T.: 6 hr (slow cooking)

M.C.: Slow cooking

SERVINGS: 4

INGR.:

4 chicken thighs, boneless and skinless

1 onion, chopped

2 garlic cloves, minced

1 can (14 oz) diced tomatoes

1 can (4 oz) green chilies

4 cups chicken broth

1 tsp cumin

1 tsp chili powder

1 tsp salt

½ tsp black pepper

1 cup frozen corn

Fresh cilantro and lime wedges, for garnish

PROCEDURE:

Place chicken thighs, onion, garlic, diced tomatoes, green chilies, chicken broth, cumin, chili powder, salt, and pepper in a slow cooker.

Cook on low for 6 hours or on high for 3 hours.

Remove chicken, shred it, then return it to the soup. Add corn and heat for an additional 30 minutes.

Serve garnished with fresh cilantro and lime wedges.

TIPS:

Add a can of rinsed and drained black beans for extra fiber and protein.

Top with crispy tortilla strips, diced avocado, and a dollop of sour cream or Greek yogurt for serving.

N.V.: Calories: 320, Fat: 12g, Carbs: 27g, Protein: 28g, Sugar: 5g

9.3 BEEF AND BARLEY STEW

1. TRADITIONAL BEEF AND BARLEY STEW

P.T.: 20 min

C.T.: 1 hr 30 min

M.C.: Simmering

SERVINGS: 6

INGR.:

1 lb lean beef stew meat, cut into cubes

2 Tbsp olive oil

1 onion, chopped

2 carrots, peeled and diced

2 celery stalks, diced

2 garlic cloves, minced

6 cups low-sodium beef broth

1 cup barley

1 tsp dried thyme

1 bay leaf

Salt and pepper to taste

Fresh parsley, chopped (for garnish)

PROCEDURE:

In a large pot, heat 1 tablespoon of olive oil over medium-high heat. Brown the beef cubes in batches, then set aside. In the same pot, add the remaining olive oil, onion, carrots, celery, and garlic, sautéing until softened. Return the beef to the pot, add beef broth, barley, thyme, and bay leaf. Season with salt and pepper.

Bring to a boil, then reduce heat to low and simmer, covered, for about 1 hour and 30 minutes, or until the beef and barley are tender. Remove the bay leaf, adjust seasoning, and serve garnished with fresh parsley.

TIPS:

For a thicker stew, remove a portion of the cooked barley and vegetables, blend, and then stir back into the stew. Add a splash of red wine with the beef broth for added depth of flavor.

N.V.: Calories: 350, Fat: 10g, Carbs: 40g, Protein: 25g, Sugar: 4g

---

2. MUSHROOM AND BEEF BARLEY STEW

P.T.: 20 min

C.T.: 1 hr 30 min

M.C.: Simmering

SERVINGS: 6

INGR.:

1 lb lean beef stew meat, cut into pieces

1 Tbsp olive oil

1 onion, diced

2 garlic cloves, minced

8 oz mushrooms, sliced

2 carrots, diced

6 cups low-sodium beef broth

1 cup barley

1 tsp dried rosemary

Salt and pepper to taste

Fresh thyme, for garnish

PROCEDURE:

Brown the beef in a large pot with olive oil over medium-high heat, then set aside. In the same pot, sauté onion, garlic, and mushrooms until softened. Add the beef back to the pot along with carrots, beef broth, barley, and rosemary. Season with salt and pepper. Bring to a boil, then reduce heat and simmer, covered, until the beef and barley are tender, about 1 hour and 30 minutes. Serve hot, garnished with fresh thyme.

TIPS:

For a more robust mushroom flavor, use a mix of wild mushrooms. A dash of Worcestershire sauce can be added to the stew for extra umami flavor.

N.V.: Calories: 360, Fat: 10g, Carbs: 42g, Protein: 26g, Sugar: 5g

3. SLOW-COOKER BEEF AND BARLEY STEW

P.T.: 20 min

C.T.: 8 hr (slow cooking)

M.C.: Slow cooking

SERVINGS: 6

INGR.:

1 lb lean beef stew meat, cut into cubes

1 Tbsp olive oil

1 large onion, chopped

2 carrots, peeled and sliced

2 celery stalks, sliced

3 garlic cloves, minced

6 cups low-sodium beef broth

1 cup pearl barley

1 tsp dried thyme

1 bay leaf

Salt and pepper to taste

Fresh parsley, for garnish

PROCEDURE:

In a skillet, heat olive oil over medium-high heat. Brown the beef cubes, then transfer to the slow cooker.

Add onion, carrots, celery, garlic, beef broth, barley, thyme, and bay leaf to the slow cooker. Season with salt and pepper.

Cook on low for 8 hours, or until the beef and barley are tender.

Adjust seasoning, remove the bay leaf, and serve garnished with fresh parsley.

TIPS:

For a richer flavor, deglaze the skillet with a splash of wine after browning the beef and add the juices to the slow cooker.

Stir in some fresh spinach or kale during the last 30 minutes of cooking for added greens.

N.V.: Calories: 330, Fat: 9g, Carbs: 39g, Protein: 27g, Sugar: 5g

4. BEEF AND BARLEY STEW WITH ROOT VEGETABLES

P.T.: 20 min

C.T.: 2 hr

M.C.: Simmering

SERVINGS: 6

INGR.:

1 lb lean beef stew meat, cut into cubes

2 Tbsp olive oil

1 onion, chopped

2 carrots, peeled and cubed

2 parsnips, peeled and cubed

1 turnip, peeled and cubed

3 garlic cloves, minced

6 cups low-sodium beef broth

1 cup barley

1 tsp dried thyme

Salt and pepper to taste

Fresh parsley, for garnish

PROCEDURE:

Heat olive oil in a large pot and brown the beef, then set aside.

In the same pot, sauté onion, carrots, parsnips, turnip, and garlic until slightly softened.

Return the beef to the pot, add broth, barley,

and thyme. Season with salt and pepper. Bring to a boil, then reduce heat to low and simmer, covered, until the vegetables and barley are tender, about 1.5 to 2 hours. Serve hot, garnished with fresh parsley.

TIPS:

Roasting the root vegetables before adding them to the stew can enhance their sweetness and depth of flavor.

A splash of balsamic vinegar or tomato paste can be added to the stew for extra richness.

N.V.: Calories: 350, Fat: 10g, Carbs: 45g, Protein: 28g, Sugar: 6g

---

5. SPICY BEEF AND BARLEY STEW

P.T.: 20 min

C.T.: 1 hr 30 min

M.C.: Simmering

SERVINGS: 6

INGR.:

1 lb lean beef stew meat, cut into cubes

1 Tbsp olive oil

1 onion, chopped

2 garlic cloves, minced

2 jalapeños, seeded and diced

1 tsp smoked paprika

1 tsp cumin

6 cups low-sodium beef broth

1 cup barley

1 can (14 oz) diced tomatoes

Salt and pepper to taste

Chopped cilantro, for garnish

PROCEDURE:

Heat olive oil in a large pot, brown the beef, then remove and set aside.

Add onion, garlic, jalapeños, smoked paprika, and cumin to the pot, cooking until onions are soft.

Return the beef to the pot, add beef broth, barley, and diced tomatoes. Season with salt and pepper.

Simmer covered, until the barley and beef are tender, about 1.5 hours.

Serve hot, garnished with chopped cilantro.

TIPS:

Adjust the amount of jalapeños according to your spice preference.

A splash of lime juice added before serving can brighten the flavors.

N.V.: Calories: 340, Fat: 9g, Carbs: 41g, Protein: 29g, Sugar: 7g

---

6. HERBED BEEF AND BARLEY STEW

P.T.: 20 min

C.T.: 2 hr

M.C.: Simmering

SERVINGS: 6

INGR.:

1 lb lean beef stew meat, cut into cubes

2 Tbsp olive oil

1 large onion, chopped

3 cloves garlic, minced

1 cup barley

6 cups low-sodium beef broth

2 carrots, diced

2 stalks celery, diced

1 tsp dried rosemary

1 tsp dried thyme

Salt and pepper to taste

Fresh parsley, chopped (for garnish)

PROCEDURE:

In a large pot, heat olive oil and brown the beef on all sides. Remove and set aside.

Add onion, garlic, carrots, and celery to the pot, cooking until vegetables are tender.

Stir in barley, beef broth, rosemary, thyme, and return the beef to the pot. Season with salt and pepper.

Bring to a boil, then reduce heat to low and simmer, covered, for about 2 hours or until the beef and barley are tender.

Adjust seasoning and serve garnished with fresh parsley.

TIPS:

For a richer stew, deglaze the pot with a splash of red wine after browning the beef and sautéing the vegetables.

A handful of fresh spinach or kale can be stirred in at the end of cooking for added nutrition.

N.V.: Calories: 330, Fat: 9g, Carbs: 40g, Protein: 28g, Sugar: 4g

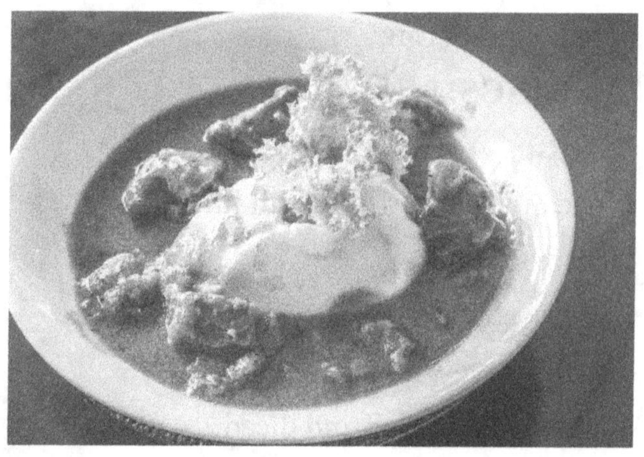

CHAPTER 10: VEGETARIAN FAVORITES

10.1 STUFFED BELL PEPPERS

1. CLASSIC VEGETARIAN STUFFED BELL PEPPERS

P.T.: 20 min

C.T.: 30 min

M.C.: Baking

SERVINGS: 4

INGR.:

4 large bell peppers, tops cut off and seeds removed

1 cup cooked quinoa

1 can (15 oz) black beans, rinsed and drained

1 cup corn kernels

1 cup tomato sauce

1 tsp cumin

1 tsp paprika

1 tsp garlic powder

Salt and pepper to taste

1 cup shredded low-fat cheese

Fresh cilantro, for garnish

PROCEDURE:

Preheat the oven to 375°F (190°C).

In a bowl, mix quinoa, black beans, corn, tomato sauce, cumin, paprika, garlic powder, salt, and pepper.

Stuff each bell pepper with the quinoa mixture and place them in a baking dish.

Cover with foil and bake for 25 minutes.

Remove foil, top each pepper with cheese, and bake for an additional 5 minutes or until cheese is melted.

Garnish with fresh cilantro before serving.

TIPS:

For added protein, mix in some chopped nuts or seeds with the quinoa filling.

Play with different colors of bell peppers to make the dish more visually appealing.

N.V.: Calories: 280, Fat: 5g, Carbs: 45g, Protein: 15g, Sugar: 8g

2. MEDITERRANEAN STUFFED BELL PEPPERS

P.T.: 20 min

C.T.: 30 min

M.C.: Baking

SERVINGS: 4

INGR.:

4 large bell peppers, halved and seeded

1 cup cooked farro or bulgur wheat

1 can (15 oz) chickpeas, rinsed and drained

1 cup chopped spinach

½ cup crumbled feta cheese

1 cup diced tomatoes

1 tsp oregano

1 tsp thyme

Salt and pepper to taste

Olive oil for drizzling

PROCEDURE:

Preheat the oven to 375°F (190°C).

Combine farro, chickpeas, spinach, feta, tomatoes, oregano, thyme, salt, and pepper in a bowl.

Fill each bell pepper half with the mixture and place them in a baking dish.

Drizzle with olive oil, cover with foil, and bake for 20 minutes.

Uncover and bake for an additional 10 minutes or until peppers are tender and filling is heated through.

TIPS:

Add some pine nuts or olives to the stuffing for a crunchy texture and extra flavor.

Drizzle with balsamic reduction before serving for a gourmet touch.

N.V.: Calories: 300, Fat: 9g, Carbs: 45g, Protein: 14g, Sugar: 9g

---

3. MEXICAN-STYLE STUFFED BELL PEPPERS

P.T.: 25 min

C.T.: 35 min

M.C.: Baking

SERVINGS: 4

INGR.:

4 large bell peppers, tops cut off and seeds removed

1 cup cooked brown rice

1 can (15 oz) black beans, rinsed and drained

1 cup corn kernels

1 cup salsa

1 tsp chili powder

1 tsp cumin

Salt and pepper to taste

1 cup shredded low-fat cheddar cheese

Fresh cilantro and avocado slices, for garnish

PROCEDURE:

Preheat oven to 375°F (190°C).

In a bowl, combine brown rice, black beans, corn, salsa, chili powder, cumin, salt, and pepper.

Stuff the mixture into the bell peppers and place them in a baking dish.

Cover with foil and bake for 30 minutes.

Remove foil, top peppers with cheddar cheese, and bake uncovered for an additional 5 minutes or until cheese is melted.

Garnish with cilantro and avocado slices before serving.

TIPS:

Enhance the filling with diced jalapeños or green chilies for extra heat.

Serve with a dollop of low-fat sour cream or Greek yogurt.

N.V.: Calories: 320, Fat: 8g, Carbs: 50g, Protein: 16g, Sugar: 10g

---

4. ITALIAN STUFFED BELL PEPPERS

P.T.: 20 min

C.T.: 40 min

M.C.: Baking

SERVINGS: 4

INGR.:

4 large bell peppers, halved and deseeded

1 cup cooked orzo or small pasta

1 cup marinara sauce

1 cup ricotta cheese

1 egg, beaten

1 tsp garlic powder

1 tsp dried basil

Salt and pepper to taste

1 cup shredded mozzarella cheese

Fresh basil, for garnish

PROCEDURE:

Preheat oven to 375°F (190°C).

Mix orzo, marinara sauce, ricotta cheese, egg, garlic powder, dried basil, salt, and pepper in a bowl.

Stuff the bell pepper halves with the pasta mixture, and place in a baking dish.

Cover with foil and bake for 30 minutes.

Uncover, top with mozzarella cheese, and bake for an additional 10 minutes or until cheese is bubbly and golden.

Garnish with fresh basil leaves before serving.

TIPS:

Add some cooked ground turkey or vegetarian crumble for a protein boost.

Replace orzo with quinoa for a gluten-free option.

N.V.: Calories: 330, Fat: 15g, Carbs: 35g, Protein: 18g, Sugar: 8g

5. ASIAN-STYLE STUFFED BELL PEPPERS

P.T.: 20 min

C.T.: 30 min

M.C.: Baking

SERVINGS: 4

INGR.:

4 large bell peppers, tops cut off and seeds removed

1 cup cooked jasmine rice

1 cup shredded cabbage

1 cup shredded carrots

½ cup chopped green onions

1 Tbsp soy sauce

1 tsp sesame oil

1 tsp ginger, grated

1 garlic clove, minced

2 Tbsp hoisin sauce

Sesame seeds and additional green onions, for garnish

PROCEDURE:

Preheat oven to 375°F (190°C).

In a bowl, combine jasmine rice, cabbage, carrots, green onions, soy sauce, sesame oil, ginger, garlic, and hoisin sauce.

Fill the bell peppers with the rice mixture and place them in a baking dish.

Cover with foil and bake for 25 minutes.

Uncover and bake for an additional 5 minutes.

Garnish with sesame seeds and green onions before serving.

TIPS:

Add cooked shrimp or tofu to the filling for extra protein.

Drizzle with a little sriracha or sweet chili sauce for a spicy kick.

N.V.: Calories: 270, Fat: 5g, Carbs: 50g, Protein: 8g, Sugar: 12g

P.T.: 25 min

C.T.: 35 min

M.C.: Baking

SERVINGS: 4

INGR.:

4 large bell peppers, halved and deseeded

1 cup cooked couscous

1 can (15 oz) chickpeas, rinsed and drained

1 cup chopped spinach

½ cup crumbled feta cheese

1 cup diced tomatoes

1 tsp dried oregano

Salt and pepper to taste

Olive oil for drizzling

Fresh dill, for garnish

PROCEDURE:

Preheat oven to 375°F (190°C).

Combine couscous, chickpeas, spinach, feta cheese, tomatoes, oregano, salt, and pepper in a bowl.

Fill bell pepper halves with the couscous mixture, place in a baking dish, and drizzle with olive oil.

Cover with foil and bake for 30 minutes.

Uncover and bake for an additional 5 minutes or until peppers are tender.

Garnish with fresh dill before serving.

TIPS:

Add some olives or artichoke hearts to the filling for more Mediterranean flavors.

Drizzle with tzatziki sauce before serving for added creaminess and flavor.

N.V.: Calories: 290, Fat: 9g, Carbs: 42g, Protein: 12g, Sugar: 9g

10.2 EGGPLANT AND CHICKPEA CURRY

1. CLASSIC EGGPLANT AND CHICKPEA CURRY

P.T.: 15 min

C.T.: 30 min

M.C.: Sautéing and simmering

SERVINGS: 4

INGR.:

2 medium eggplants, cubed

1 can (15 oz) chickpeas, drained and rinsed

2 Tbsp olive oil

1 large onion, chopped

2 garlic cloves, minced

1 Tbsp ginger, grated

2 tsp ground cumin

2 tsp ground coriander

1 tsp turmeric

1 tsp paprika

1 can (14 oz) diced tomatoes

1 can (14 oz) coconut milk

Salt and pepper to taste

Fresh cilantro, for garnish

PROCEDURE:

Heat olive oil in a large pan over medium heat. Sauté onion, garlic, and ginger until onion is translucent.

Add cumin, coriander, turmeric, and paprika, cooking for another minute until fragrant.

Stir in eggplant and chickpeas, coating them

with the spices.

Add diced tomatoes and coconut milk, season with salt and pepper.

Bring to a boil, then reduce heat and simmer for 20-25 minutes, until eggplant is tender.

Garnish with fresh cilantro and serve with rice or naan.

TIPS:

Salt the eggplant cubes and let them sit for 10 minutes before cooking to draw out moisture and bitterness.

Add a splash of lime juice before serving to enhance the flavors.

N.V.: Calories: 350, Fat: 18g, Carbs: 40g, Protein: 9g, Sugar: 14g

<hr>

2. SPICY EGGPLANT AND CHICKPEA CURRY

P.T.: 15 min

C.T.: 30 min

M.C.: Sautéing and simmering

SERVINGS: 4

INGR.:

2 medium eggplants, cubed

1 can (15 oz) chickpeas, drained and rinsed

2 Tbsp vegetable oil

1 onion, finely chopped

3 garlic cloves, minced

1 Tbsp ginger, grated

1 green chili, finely chopped

1 Tbsp curry powder

1 tsp garam masala

1 can (14 oz) diced tomatoes

1 cup vegetable broth

Salt to taste

Fresh cilantro and sliced chilies, for garnish

PROCEDURE:

In a large pot, heat oil over medium heat. Add onion, garlic, ginger, and green chili; sauté until onion is soft.

Stir in curry powder and garam masala, cooking until fragrant.

Add eggplant and chickpeas, ensuring they are well coated with the spice mixture.

Pour in diced tomatoes and vegetable broth, season with salt.

Simmer for 25-30 minutes, until eggplant is tender and flavors meld.

Serve garnished with cilantro and sliced chilies, accompanied by basmati rice or flatbread.

TIPS:

Adjust the heat by increasing or reducing the amount of green chili.

A splash of coconut milk can be added for a creamier texture.

N.V.: Calories: 330, Fat: 10g, Carbs: 50g, Protein: 11g, Sugar: 13g

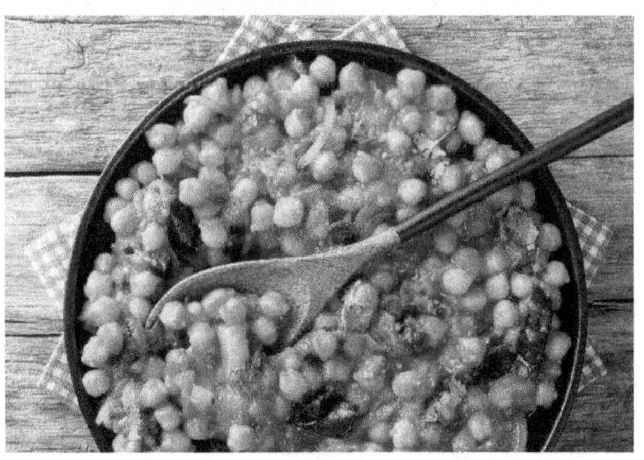

3. Eggplant and Chickpea Curry with Spinach

P.T.: 20 min

C.T.: 40 min

M.C.: Sautéing and simmering

SERVINGS: 4

INGR.:

2 medium eggplants, cubed

1 can (15 oz) chickpeas, drained and rinsed

2 Tbsp olive oil

1 onion, diced

2 garlic cloves, minced

1 Tbsp fresh ginger, minced

2 tsp curry powder

1 tsp ground turmeric

1 can (14 oz) diced tomatoes

1 can (14 oz) coconut milk

3 cups fresh spinach leaves

Salt and pepper to taste

Fresh cilantro, for garnish

PROCEDURE:

Heat olive oil in a large pot over medium heat.

Sauté onion, garlic, and ginger until onion is soft.

Add curry powder and turmeric, stir for 1 minute until fragrant.

Incorporate eggplant and chickpeas, cooking for a few minutes to blend the flavors.

Mix in diced tomatoes and coconut milk, season with salt and pepper, and bring to a simmer.

Cover and cook for 30 minutes, or until eggplant is tender.

Stir in spinach until wilted. Adjust seasoning and serve garnished with cilantro.

TIPS:

For a thicker curry, mash some of the chickpeas before adding them to the pot.

Lemon juice can be added at the end of cooking for a tangy finish.

N.V.: Calories: 360, Fat: 20g, Carbs: 42g, Protein: 11g, Sugar: 14g

4. Eggplant, Chickpea, and Sweet Potato Curry

P.T.: 20 min

C.T.: 40 min

M.C.: Sautéing and simmering

SERVINGS: 4

INGR.:

1 large eggplant, cubed

1 large sweet potato, cubed

1 can (15 oz) chickpeas, drained and rinsed

2 Tbsp vegetable oil

1 large onion, chopped

3 garlic cloves, minced

1 Tbsp grated ginger

2 tsp curry powder

1 tsp ground cumin

1 can (14 oz) diced tomatoes

1 can (14 oz) coconut milk

Salt and pepper to taste

Fresh cilantro, for garnish

PROCEDURE:

In a large pot, heat oil over medium heat.

Sauté onion, garlic, and ginger until soft. Add curry powder and cumin, cook until fragrant. Mix in eggplant, sweet potato, and chickpeas. Pour in diced tomatoes and coconut milk, season with salt and pepper, and bring to a simmer. Cook covered for 35-40 minutes, or until vegetables are tender. Serve garnished with cilantro, alongside rice or naan.

TIPS:

Roasting the eggplant and sweet potato beforehand can add a smoky depth to the curry.

Add a pinch of chili flakes for a spicy kick.

N.V.: Calories: 380, Fat: 18g, Carbs: 50g, Protein: 10g, Sugar: 16g

---

5. EGGPLANT AND CHICKPEA THAI GREEN CURRY

P.T.: 15 min

C.T.: 30 min

M.C.: Sautéing and simmering

SERVINGS: 4

INGR.:

2 medium eggplants, cubed

1 can (15 oz) chickpeas, drained and rinsed

1 Tbsp coconut oil

2 Tbsp green curry paste

1 can (14 oz) coconut milk

1 red bell pepper, sliced

1 zucchini, sliced

1 Tbsp fish sauce (or soy sauce for a vegan option)

1 tsp brown sugar

Basil leaves, for garnish

PROCEDURE:

In a large pot, heat coconut oil over medium heat. Stir in green curry paste and cook for 1 minute.

Add eggplant and cook for 5 minutes, stirring occasionally.

Pour in coconut milk, chickpeas, bell pepper, zucchini, fish sauce, and brown sugar.

Bring to a boil, then reduce heat and simmer for 20 minutes, or until vegetables are tender. Garnish with basil leaves and serve with steamed jasmine rice.

TIPS:

Adjust the amount of curry paste to suit your taste for spiciness.

Lime juice can be added at the end for an extra zesty flavor.

N.V.: Calories: 330, Fat: 15g, Carbs: 44g, Protein: 9g, Sugar: 15g

---

6. MOROCCAN EGGPLANT AND CHICKPEA STEW

P.T.: 20 min

C.T.: 45 min

M.C.: Sautéing and simmering

SERVINGS: 4

INGR.:

2 medium eggplants, cubed

1 can (15 oz) chickpeas, drained and rinsed

2 Tbsp olive oil

1 onion, diced

3 garlic cloves, minced

1 Tbsp ground cumin

1 tsp ground cinnamon

1 tsp paprika

½ tsp ground ginger

1 can (14 oz) crushed tomatoes

2 cups vegetable broth

Salt and pepper to taste

Fresh mint, for garnish

PROCEDURE:

Heat olive oil in a large pot. Sauté onion and garlic until translucent.

Add cumin, cinnamon, paprika, and ginger, cooking until aromatic.

Stir in eggplant and chickpeas, coating them with the spices.

Add crushed tomatoes and vegetable broth, season with salt and pepper, and bring to a simmer.

Cover and cook for 40 minutes, or until eggplant is tender.

Serve hot, garnished with fresh mint, alongside couscous or flatbread.

TIPS:

For a touch of sweetness, add a handful of raisins or dried apricots to the stew.

Toast some almonds or pine nuts and sprinkle on top before serving for added crunch.

N.V.: Calories: 310, Fat: 12g, Carbs: 46g, Protein: 10g, Sugar: 18g

10.3 ZUCCHINI AND TOMATO PASTA

1. CLASSIC ZUCCHINI AND TOMATO PASTA

P.T.: 10 min

C.T.: 20 min

M.C.: Boiling and sautéing

SERVINGS: 4

INGR.:

8 oz whole wheat pasta

2 Tbsp olive oil

2 medium zucchinis, sliced

2 garlic cloves, minced

2 cups cherry tomatoes, halved

1 tsp dried basil

Salt and pepper to taste

Grated Parmesan cheese, for serving

Fresh basil leaves, for garnish

PROCEDURE:

Cook pasta according to package instructions until al dente, then drain and set aside. In a large pan, heat olive oil over medium heat. Sauté garlic until fragrant, then add zucchini, cooking until slightly tender. Add cherry tomatoes and dried basil, cooking until tomatoes are soft. Toss the cooked pasta with the zucchini and tomato mixture. Season with salt and pepper. Serve topped with grated Parmesan and garnished with fresh basil.

TIPS:

For a richer flavor, add a splash of white wine to the zucchini and tomato mixture while cooking. Roasted pine nuts or walnuts can be sprinkled on top for added crunch.

2. MEDITERRANEAN ZUCCHINI AND TOMATO PASTA

P.T.: 15 min

C.T.: 20 min

M.C.: Boiling and sautéing

SERVINGS: 4

INGR.:

8 oz whole grain penne pasta

2 Tbsp olive oil

2 medium zucchinis, diced

3 garlic cloves, minced

1 cup cherry tomatoes, halved

½ cup black olives, sliced

½ cup feta cheese, crumbled

1 tsp dried oregano

Salt and pepper to taste

Fresh parsley, chopped, for garnish

PROCEDURE:

Cook penne pasta in boiling water according to package directions until al dente, then drain.

Heat olive oil in a large skillet over medium heat. Add garlic and zucchini, sautéing until zucchini is tender.

Stir in cherry tomatoes and olives, cooking until tomatoes are just softened.

Mix in the cooked pasta, oregano, and feta cheese. Season with salt and pepper.

Serve garnished with chopped parsley.

TIPS:

A splash of lemon juice can be added for a citrusy zest.

For added protein, consider tossing in some chickpeas or grilled chicken strips.

N.V.: Calories: 350, Fat: 15g, Carbs: 45g, Protein: 12g, Sugar: 7g

N.V.: Calories: 320, Fat: 10g, Carbs: 48g, Protein: 12g, Sugar: 6g

3. CREAMY ZUCCHINI AND TOMATO PASTA

P.T.: 10 min

C.T.: 20 min

M.C.: Boiling and sautéing

SERVINGS: 4

INGR.:

8 oz whole wheat spaghetti

2 Tbsp olive oil

2 medium zucchinis, spiralized or thinly sliced

1 small onion, finely chopped

2 garlic cloves, minced

1 cup cherry tomatoes, halved

1/2 cup light cream or coconut milk

Salt and pepper to taste

Fresh basil, for garnish

Grated Parmesan cheese, optional, for serving

PROCEDURE:

Cook spaghetti according to package instructions until al dente; drain and set aside.

In a large pan, heat olive oil over medium heat. Add onion and garlic, sauté until translucent.

Add spiralized zucchini and cook until tender, about 5 minutes.

Stir in cherry tomatoes and cook until just softened.

Add cream or coconut milk to the pan, stirring to combine. Season with salt and pepper.

Toss in the cooked spaghetti, mixing until evenly coated.

Serve garnished with fresh basil and, if desired, Parmesan cheese.

TIPS:

For a vegan option, use coconut milk and vegan Parmesan cheese.

Add red pepper flakes for a spicy kick.

N.V.: Calories: 350, Fat: 12g, Carbs: 52g, Protein: 10g, Sugar: 8g

4. ZUCCHINI AND TOMATO PASTA WITH PESTO

P.T.: 15 min

C.T.: 15 min

M.C.: Boiling and sautéing

SERVINGS: 4

INGR.:

8 oz whole wheat fusilli pasta

2 Tbsp olive oil

2 medium zucchinis, cubed

2 cups cherry tomatoes, halved

1/2 cup homemade or store-bought pesto

Salt and pepper to taste

Fresh basil leaves, for garnish

Grated Parmesan cheese, for serving

PROCEDURE:

Cook fusilli pasta in boiling water until al dente; drain and set aside.

In a large skillet, heat olive oil over medium heat. Add zucchinis and sauté until just tender.

Add cherry tomatoes and cook until they start to soften.

Reduce heat and stir in pesto, mixing well with the vegetables.

Toss the pesto mixture with the cooked pasta, season with salt and pepper.

Serve garnished with basil leaves and Parmesan cheese.

TIPS:

To enhance the dish, add toasted pine nuts or walnuts before serving.

For added protein, mix in some white beans or grilled chicken strips.

N.V.: Calories: 400, Fat: 18g, Carbs: 50g, Protein: 12g, Sugar: 6g

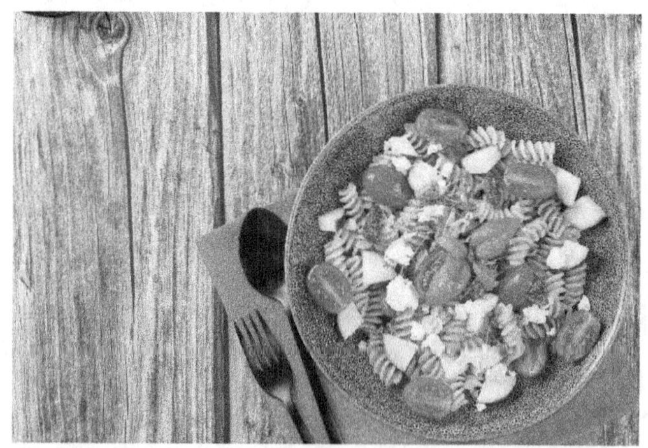

5. ZUCCHINI AND TOMATO PASTA WITH LEMON AND HERBS

P.T.: 10 min

C.T.: 20 min

M.C.: Boiling and sautéing

SERVINGS: 4

INGR.:

8 oz whole wheat angel hair pasta

2 Tbsp olive oil

2 medium zucchinis, thinly sliced

2 cups grape tomatoes, halved

2 garlic cloves, minced

Zest and juice of 1 lemon

1 tsp dried Italian herbs

Salt and pepper to taste

Fresh parsley, chopped, for garnish

PROCEDURE:

Cook angel hair pasta according to package instructions until al dente; drain and set aside.

In a large skillet, heat olive oil over medium heat. Sauté zucchini and garlic until zucchini is slightly tender.

Add tomatoes, lemon zest, and juice, cooking until tomatoes are just softened.

Stir in Italian herbs, and season with salt and pepper.

Toss the vegetable mixture with the cooked pasta.

Serve garnished with chopped parsley.

TIPS:

Add capers or olives for a briny flavor.

A sprinkle of red pepper flakes can add a spicy element to the dish.

N.V.: Calories: 330, Fat: 10g, Carbs: 53g, Protein: 11g, Sugar: 7g

6. RUSTIC ZUCCHINI, TOMATO, AND BELL PEPPER PASTA

P.T.: 15 min

C.T.: 25 min

M.C.: Boiling and sautéing

SERVINGS: 4

INGR.:

8 oz whole wheat penne pasta

2 Tbsp olive oil

1 medium zucchini, diced

1 medium yellow squash, diced

1 red bell pepper, diced

2 cups cherry tomatoes, halved

3 garlic cloves, minced

1 tsp dried basil

1 tsp dried oregano

Salt and pepper to taste

Fresh basil, for garnish

Shaved Parmesan cheese, for serving

PROCEDURE:

Cook penne pasta according to package instructions until al dente; drain and set aside.

In a large skillet, heat olive oil over medium heat. Sauté zucchini, yellow squash, bell pepper, and garlic until tender.

Add cherry tomatoes, basil, and oregano, cooking until tomatoes are soft.

Season with salt and pepper, then toss the vegetable mixture with the cooked pasta.

Serve garnished with fresh basil and shaved Parmesan cheese.

TIPS:

For a smoky flavor, grill the vegetables before adding them to the pasta.

Incorporate a splash of white wine while sautéing the vegetables for added depth.

N.V.: Calories: 340, Fat: 10g, Carbs: 54g, Protein: 12g, Sugar: 8g

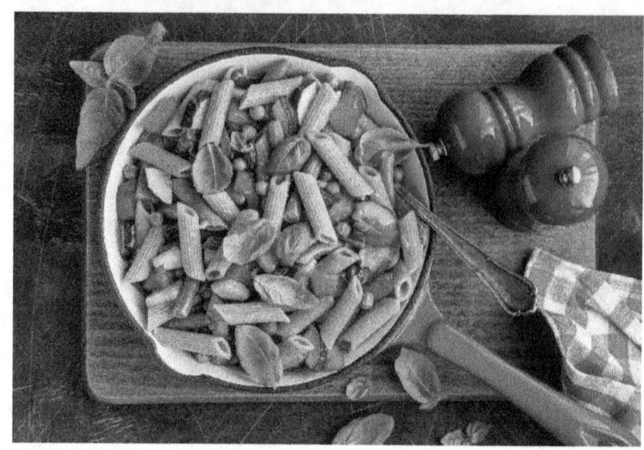

CHAPTER 11: QUICK AND EASY DASH MEALS
11.1 FIFTEEN-MINUTE STIR-FRY VEGETABLES WITH BROWN RICE

1. CLASSIC VEGETABLE STIR-FRY WITH BROWN RICE

P.T.: 5 min

C.T.: 10 min

M.C.: Stir-frying

SERVINGS: 4

INGR.:

2 cups cooked brown rice

1 Tbsp olive oil

1 red bell pepper, sliced

1 yellow bell pepper, sliced

1 zucchini, sliced

1 carrot, julienned

1 cup broccoli florets

2 garlic cloves, minced

2 Tbsp soy sauce (low sodium)

1 tsp sesame oil

Salt and pepper to taste

Sesame seeds, for garnish

PROCEDURE:

Heat olive oil in a large wok or skillet over high heat.

Add garlic, bell peppers, zucchini, carrot, and broccoli, stir-frying until just tender, about 5 minutes.

Stir in soy sauce and sesame oil, tossing the vegetables to coat evenly. Season with salt and pepper.

Serve the stir-fried vegetables over cooked brown rice, sprinkled with sesame seeds.

TIPS:

Keep the vegetables moving in the pan to prevent burning and ensure even cooking.

For added protein, include tofu, chicken, or shrimp in the stir-fry.

N.V.: Calories: 220, Fat: 5g, Carbs: 38g, Protein: 6g, Sugar: 5g

2. SPICY THAI VEGETABLE STIR-FRY WITH BROWN RICE

P.T.: 5 min

C.T.: 10 min

M.C.: Stir-frying

SERVINGS: 4

INGR.:

2 cups cooked brown rice

1 Tbsp coconut oil

1 small red onion, sliced

1 red bell pepper, sliced

1 cup snap peas

1 cup baby corn

1 carrot, julienned

2 Tbsp Thai red curry paste

1 can (14 oz) coconut milk

Salt to taste

Fresh basil leaves, for garnish

PROCEDURE:

Heat coconut oil in a wok over medium-high heat.

Sauté onion, bell pepper, snap peas, baby

corn, and carrot until slightly tender, about 5 minutes.

Stir in Thai red curry paste and coconut milk, mixing well. Cook for another 5 minutes until the sauce thickens slightly.

Serve the spicy vegetable stir-fry over brown rice, garnished with fresh basil leaves.

TIPS:

Adjust the amount of curry paste to control the spice level.

Add tofu or chicken for a protein boost.

N.V.: Calories: 300, Fat: 12g, Carbs: 42g, Protein: 7g, Sugar: 6g

---

3. GINGER BEEF STIR-FRY WITH BROWN RICE

P.T.: 5 min

C.T.: 10 min

M.C.: Stir-frying

SERVINGS: 4

INGR.:

2 cups cooked brown rice

1 Tbsp vegetable oil

1 lb lean beef, thinly sliced

1 red bell pepper, julienned

1 green bell pepper, julienned

2 cups broccoli florets

2 tsp fresh ginger, minced

2 garlic cloves, minced

3 Tbsp low-sodium soy sauce

1 Tbsp oyster sauce

1 tsp sesame oil

Salt and pepper to taste

Green onions, sliced, for garnish

PROCEDURE:

Heat oil in a large wok or skillet over high heat.

Add beef slices, stirring until browned and nearly cooked through, about 3 minutes.

Add bell peppers, broccoli, ginger, and garlic, stir-frying until vegetables are tender-crisp, about 5 minutes.

Mix in soy sauce, oyster sauce, and sesame oil, stirring to coat the beef and vegetables evenly. Season with salt and pepper.

Serve the ginger beef stir-fry over cooked brown rice, garnished with green onions.

TIPS:

Ensure the beef is sliced against the grain for tender, easy-to-eat pieces.

A splash of rice wine vinegar can be added for extra tanginess.

N.V.: Calories: 340, Fat: 10g, Carbs: 38g, Protein: 25g, Sugar: 5g

---

4. TOFU AND VEGETABLE STIR-FRY WITH BROWN RICE

P.T.: 5 min

C.T.: 10 min

M.C.: Stir-frying

SERVINGS: 4

INGR.:

2 cups cooked brown rice

1 Tbsp sesame oil

14 oz firm tofu, drained, pressed, and cubed

1 cup sliced mushrooms

1 red bell pepper, sliced

1 zucchini, sliced

1 cup snow peas

2 Tbsp low-sodium soy sauce

1 Tbsp hoisin sauce

1 tsp ground ginger

Salt and pepper to taste

Sesame seeds and chopped cilantro, for garnish

PROCEDURE:

Heat sesame oil in a large wok or skillet over medium-high heat.

Add tofu cubes, stir-frying until golden brown on all sides, about 5 minutes.

Add mushrooms, bell pepper, zucchini, and snow peas, cooking until vegetables are tender, about 5 minutes.

Stir in soy sauce, hoisin sauce, and ground ginger, coating the tofu and vegetables evenly. Season with salt and pepper.

Serve the tofu and vegetable stir-fry over brown rice, sprinkled with sesame seeds and cilantro.

TIPS:

For extra flavor, marinate the tofu in a mixture of soy sauce, ginger, and garlic before stir-frying.

Add a splash of water or vegetable broth if the stir-fry is too dry or to help deglaze the pan.

N.V.: Calories: 320, Fat: 12g, Carbs: 40g, Protein: 16g, Sugar: 6g

11.2 ONE-POT CHICKEN FAJITAS

1. CLASSIC ONE-POT CHICKEN FAJITAS

P.T.: 10 min

C.T.: 20 min

M.C.: Sautéing

SERVINGS: 4

INGR.:

1 lb chicken breast, thinly sliced

1 Tbsp olive oil

1 red bell pepper, sliced

1 green bell pepper, sliced

1 onion, sliced

2 garlic cloves, minced

1 tsp chili powder

1 tsp cumin

1 tsp paprika

Salt and pepper to taste

Juice of 1 lime

Fresh cilantro, chopped, for garnish

Whole wheat tortillas, for serving

PROCEDURE:

Heat olive oil in a large skillet over medium-high heat.

Add chicken slices, cooking until browned and nearly cooked through.

Add bell peppers, onion, and garlic, sautéing until vegetables are tender.

Sprinkle with chili powder, cumin, and paprika. Season with salt and pepper.

Squeeze lime juice over the fajita mixture and

stir well.

Serve the chicken and vegetables in whole wheat tortillas, garnished with fresh cilantro.

TIPS:

For best flavor, marinate the chicken in lime juice and spices for at least 30 minutes before cooking.

Serve with avocado slices or guacamole for added creaminess.

N.V.: Calories: 300, Fat: 8g, Carbs: 25g, Protein: 30g, Sugar: 5g

---

2. SPICY ONE-POT CHICKEN FAJITAS

P.T.: 10 min

C.T.: 20 min

M.C.: Sautéing

SERVINGS: 4

INGR.:

1 lb chicken breast, thinly sliced

1 Tbsp vegetable oil

2 bell peppers (any color), sliced

1 large onion, sliced

2 tsp chipotle powder

1 tsp garlic powder

1 tsp onion powder

Salt and pepper to taste

Juice of 1 lime

Fresh cilantro, for garnish

Whole wheat tortillas, for serving

Sliced jalapeños, for garnish

PROCEDURE:

Heat oil in a large skillet over medium-high heat.

Cook chicken until it starts to brown.

Add bell peppers and onion, cooking until slightly softened.

Stir in chipotle powder, garlic powder, and onion powder. Season with salt and pepper.

Add lime juice, mixing well.

Serve in tortillas, topped with cilantro and jalapeños for extra spice.

TIPS:

Increase or decrease the amount of chipotle powder according to your spice preference.

Accompany with a side of sour cream or Greek yogurt to balance the heat.

N.V.: Calories: 320, Fat: 9g, Carbs: 27g, Protein: 32g, Sugar: 6g

---

3. ONE-POT CHICKEN FAJITAS WITH MANGO SALSA

P.T.: 15 min

C.T.: 20 min

M.C.: Sautéing

SERVINGS: 4

INGR.:

1 lb chicken breast, thinly sliced

1 Tbsp olive oil

1 red bell pepper, sliced

1 yellow bell pepper, sliced

1 onion, sliced

2 tsp taco seasoning

Salt and pepper to taste

Juice of 1 lime

For the Mango Salsa:

1 ripe mango, diced

1/4 cup red onion, finely chopped

1 jalapeño, minced (optional)

Juice of 1 lime

Salt to taste

Fresh cilantro, for garnish

Whole wheat tortillas, for serving

PROCEDURE:

In a large skillet, heat olive oil over medium-high heat. Add chicken and cook until browned.

Add bell peppers and onion, sautéing until soft. Sprinkle with taco seasoning, salt, and pepper.

Prepare the salsa by combining mango, red onion, jalapeño, lime juice, and salt in a bowl.

Squeeze lime juice over the chicken and vegetable mix, stir well.

Serve the fajitas in tortillas with a spoonful of mango salsa and garnished with cilantro.

TIPS:

For a sweeter salsa, add a bit of honey to the mango mixture.

Avocado chunks can be added to the salsa for creaminess and extra nutrients.

N.V.: Calories: 330, Fat: 9g, Carbs: 35g, Protein: 30g, Sugar: 15g

---

4. ONE-POT CREAMY CHICKEN FAJITAS

P.T.: 10 min

C.T.: 20 min

M.C.: Sautéing

SERVINGS: 4

INGR.:

1 lb chicken breast, thinly sliced

1 Tbsp olive oil

1 red bell pepper, sliced

1 green bell pepper, sliced

1 onion, sliced

1 tsp garlic powder

1 tsp onion powder

1 cup low-fat sour cream

2 Tbsp fajita seasoning

Salt and pepper to taste

Whole wheat tortillas, for serving

Chopped green onions, for garnish

PROCEDURE:

Heat olive oil in a large skillet over medium-high heat. Cook chicken until golden brown.

Add bell peppers and onion, sautéing until they are tender.

Sprinkle garlic powder, onion powder, and fajita seasoning over the chicken and vegetables. Stir well.

Lower the heat and mix in sour cream, heating through but not boiling. Season with salt and pepper.

Serve the creamy chicken fajita mixture in tortillas, garnished with green onions.

TIPS:

To thin the sauce if necessary, add a splash of

chicken broth. Add diced tomatoes to the skillet before adding sour cream for a tangy twist.

N.V.: Calories: 340, Fat: 14g, Carbs: 28g, Protein: 31g, Sugar: 7g

11.3 SHRIMP AND BROCCOLI IN GARLIC SAUCE

1. CLASSIC SHRIMP AND BROCCOLI IN GARLIC SAUCE

P.T.: 10 min

C.T.: 10 min

M.C.: Sautéing

SERVINGS: 4

INGR.:

1 lb shrimp, peeled and deveined

4 cups broccoli florets

2 Tbsp olive oil

3 garlic cloves, minced

2 Tbsp low-sodium soy sauce

1 Tbsp oyster sauce

1 tsp sesame oil

1 tsp cornstarch, dissolved in 2 Tbsp water

Salt and pepper to taste

PROCEDURE:

Heat olive oil in a large skillet over medium-high heat.

Add garlic and sauté until fragrant.

Add shrimp and cook until they turn pink, about 3 minutes.

Add broccoli, soy sauce, and oyster sauce, stirring to combine.

Stir in the cornstarch mixture and cook until the sauce thickens and broccoli is tender, about 5 minutes.

Drizzle with sesame oil and season with salt and pepper before serving.

TIPS:

Ensure not to overcook the shrimp to keep them tender.

Add a splash of chicken or vegetable broth for a saucier dish.

N.V.: Calories: 240, Fat: 10g, Carbs: 10g, Protein: 25g, Sugar: 3g

2. SPICY SHRIMP AND BROCCOLI STIR-FRY

P.T.: 10 min

C.T.: 10 min

M.C.: Stir-frying

SERVINGS: 4

INGR.:

1 lb shrimp, peeled and deveined

4 cups broccoli florets

2 Tbsp vegetable oil

1 Tbsp garlic, minced

1 Tbsp ginger, minced

2 tsp chili flakes

2 Tbsp low-sodium soy sauce

1 tsp honey

1 Tbsp rice vinegar

Salt to taste

Green onions, sliced, for garnish

PROCEDURE:

Heat oil in a wok or large skillet over high

heat. Add garlic, ginger, and chili flakes, cooking until aromatic.

Toss in shrimp and stir-fry until nearly cooked through.

Add broccoli, soy sauce, honey, and rice vinegar, stir-frying until the broccoli is crisp-tender.

Adjust seasoning with salt and garnish with green onions before serving.

TIPS:

For extra heat, increase the amount of chili flakes or add fresh sliced chilies.

Serve with brown rice or quinoa for a complete meal.

N.V.: Calories: 250, Fat: 8g, Carbs: 12g, Protein: 28g, Sugar: 5g

CHAPTER 12: 60-DAY DASH DIET MEAL PLAN

12.1 WEEK 1-4: INTRODUCTION AND GRADUAL SODIUM REDUCTION

Day	Breakfast	Snack 1	Lunch	Snack 2	Dinner
Monday	Hearty Whole-Grain Pancakes	Hummus and Veggie Sticks	Quinoa Salad with Mixed Greens	Fruit and Nut Yogurt Parfaits	Lemon and Herb Grilled Chicken
Tuesday	Spinach and Mushroom Breakfast Skillet	Fruit and Nut Yogurt Parfaits	Turkey and Avocado Wrap	Almond and Apricot Bites	Black Bean and Sweet Potato Stew
Wednesday	Banana and Walnut Oatmeal	Almond and Apricot Bites	Homemade Vegetable Soup	Hummus and Veggie Sticks	Baked Salmon with Garlic and Dijon
Thursday	Quinoa Salad with Mixed Greens	Roasted Brussels Sprouts with Almonds	Lemon and Herb Grilled Chicken	Grilled Peaches with Cinnamon	Roasted Brussels Sprouts with Almonds
Friday	Turkey and Avocado Wrap	Cauliflower Mash	Black Bean and Sweet Potato Stew	Whole Wheat Banana Bread	Cauliflower Mash
Saturday	Homemade Vegetable Soup	Quinoa and Black Bean Salad	Baked Salmon with Garlic and Dijon	Lentil and Spinach Soup	Quinoa and Black Bean Salad
Sunday	Lemon and Herb Grilled Chicken	Berry and Chia Seed Pudding	Lentil and Spinach Soup	Chicken Tortilla Soup	Beef and Barley Stew

12.2 WEEK 5-8: FULL DASH DIET INCORPORATION

Day	Breakfast	Snack 1	Lunch	Snack 2	Dinner
Monday	Stuffed Bell Peppers	Grilled Peaches with Cinnamon	Stuffed Bell Peppers	Chicken Tortilla Soup	Shrimp and Broccoli in Garlic Sauce
Tuesday	Eggplant and Chickpea Curry	Whole Wheat Banana Bread	Eggplant and Chickpea Curry	Beef and Barley Stew	Stuffed Bell Peppers
Wednesday	Zucchini and Tomato Pasta	Lentil and Spinach Soup	Zucchini and Tomato Pasta	Stuffed Bell Peppers	Eggplant and Chickpea Curry
Thursday	Fifteen-Minute Stir-Fry Vegetables with Brown Rice	Chicken Tortilla Soup	Fifteen-Minute Stir-Fry Vegetables with Brown Rice	Eggplant and Chickpea Curry	Zucchini and Tomato Pasta
Friday	One-Pot Chicken Fajitas	Beef and Barley Stew	One-Pot Chicken Fajitas	Zucchini and Tomato Pasta	Fifteen-Minute Stir-Fry Vegetables with Brown Rice
Saturday	Shrimp and Broccoli in Garlic Sauce	Stuffed Bell Peppers	Shrimp and Broccoli in Garlic Sauce	Fifteen-Minute Stir-Fry Vegetables with Brown Rice	One-Pot Chicken Fajitas
Sunday	Stuffed Bell Peppers	Eggplant and Chickpea Curry	Stuffed Bell Peppers	One-Pot Chicken Fajitas	Shrimp and Broccoli in Garlic Sauce

12.3 Tips for Sticking to Your DASH Diet Meal Plan

Embarking on the DASH diet journey is like navigating a river with gentle currents and occasional rapids. You start with enthusiasm, paddling through the calm waters of initial success and simple meal planning. However, as days pass, the currents of daily life and old eating habits can threaten to steer you off course. This journey isn't just about following a meal plan; it's about transforming your relationship with food, understanding its impact on your health, and making sustainable changes.

Imagine sitting down with a friend who has just started the DASH diet. They're feeling overwhelmed by the changes, unsure how to integrate new eating habits into their busy life. You lean in, sharing stories of those who have navigated this path successfully, blending practical advice with real-life experiences.

You recount the tale of Sarah, a single mother juggling work and family, who found success by preparing meals in advance. She dedicated Sunday afternoons to cooking and portioning out her meals for the week, ensuring that she always had DASH-friendly options at hand, even on her busiest days. Her story isn't just about meal prep; it's a testament to the power of planning and the peace of mind it brings.

Then there's Michael, a retiree who discovered the joy of fresh, local produce after starting the DASH diet. He made a ritual of visiting the farmers' market every week, turning grocery shopping into a delightful adventure rather than a chore. Michael's journey illustrates the importance of connecting with the source of your food and finding joy in the simple act of selection and preparation.

You also share insights from Emily, a college student on a tight budget, who mastered the art of shopping for affordable, DASH-friendly ingredients. She became a savvy shopper, comparing prices, opting for seasonal produce, and buying in bulk when possible. Emily's experience highlights the fact that eating healthily doesn't have to break the bank and that a little financial mindfulness can go a long way in maintaining a healthy diet.

Turning the conversation to the culinary aspect, you discuss the transformative power of herbs and spices. You describe how Mark, a former salt aficionado, learned to appreciate the robust flavors of herbs like basil, oregano, and thyme, using them to enhance his dishes without adding extra sodium. Mark's story is a culinary adventure, revealing the vast palette of flavors that can be created from simple, natural ingredients.

The journey continues with tales of social gatherings and holidays, often a challenging time for those trying to stick to a dietary plan. You recount how Jessica navigated these waters by becoming an ambassador of the DASH diet, sharing her delicious, healthy dishes at parties and family gatherings, thus turning potential obstacles into opportunities to spread awareness and inspire others.

Finally, you emphasize the importance of forgiveness and resilience, illustrated by Tom's experience. Despite occasional slip-ups, he learned not to be too hard on himself and to view each day as a new opportunity to commit to his health. Tom's story teaches the vital lesson of self-compassion and the strength found in persistence.

In weaving these narratives, you're not just providing tips for sticking to a meal plan; you're sharing a tapestry of experiences that resonate on a personal level. It's about seeing the DASH diet not as a temporary fix but as a sustainable, enjoyable way of life. This journey is filled with discovery, learning, and growth, with each person's path providing unique insights and inspiration.

As the conversation with your friend draws to a close, you remind them that the DASH diet journey is a mosaic of individual stories, including theirs. Each meal, each choice, is a step towards a healthier heart and a more vibrant life. The journey isn't always easy, but with preparation, mindfulness, and a sprinkle of creativity, it's not only achievable but deeply rewarding.

12.4 MEASUREMENT CONVERSION TABLE

Measurement	Equivalent
Volume Conversions	
1 tablespoon (tbsp)	3 teaspoons (tsp)
1 cup	16 tablespoons (tbsp)
1 fluid ounce (fl oz)	2 tablespoons (tbsp)
1 cup	8 fluid ounces (fl oz)
1 pint (pt)	2 cups
1 quart (qt)	4 cups
1 gallon (gal)	16 cups
Weight Conversions	
1 ounce (oz)	28.35 grams (g)
1 pound (lb)	16 ounces (oz)
1 kilogram (kg)	2.2 pounds (lb)
Dry Ingredient Conversions	

Measurement	Equivalent
1 cup all-purpose flour	120 grams
1 cup whole wheat flour	128 grams
1 cup granulated sugar	200 grams
1 cup brown sugar (packed)	220 grams
1 cup oats	90 grams
Liquid Ingredient Conversions	
1 cup water/milk	240 milliliters (ml)
1 cup vegetable oil	220 milliliters (ml)
1 cup honey/maple syrup	320 grams
Temperature Conversions (Oven)	
350°F	177°C
375°F	190°C
400°F	204°C
425°F	218°C

CHAPTER 13: CONCLUSION - EMBRACING A HEART-HEALTHY LIFESTYLE

13.1 CELEBRATING YOUR PROGRESS AND NEXT STEPS

As you stand on the precipice of this significant milestone, having navigated the rich landscapes of the DASH diet, it's time to pause and reflect. Reflect not just on the journey you've embarked upon but also on the transformative power of each small change you've integrated into your life. This journey was never just about food; it was about rediscovering your relationship with eating, with health, and, fundamentally, with yourself. Imagine for a moment the first steps you took. Perhaps they were tentative, filled with the quiet hope and the silent prayers of someone standing at the beginning of a path unseen. Or maybe they were bold, charged with the determination of a heart yearning for change. Regardless, those steps were yours, each one a testament to your resolve, your courage to embrace a heart-healthy lifestyle. You've learned, haven't you? About the simplicity of whole grains, the vibrancy of fruits and vegetables, the hearty sustenance provided by lean proteins, and the unexpected joy in the crunch of a fresh nut. More than that, you've learned about the hidden salt lurking in processed foods, the silent way sugar can sneak into your meals, and how, with a little awareness and creativity, these pitfalls can be avoided. But it's not just the knowledge you've gained; it's the experiences you've woven into the fabric of your life. Remember the first time you tried a recipe from the book? Maybe it was the Lemon and Herb Grilled Chicken, its aroma filling your kitchen, or perhaps the Quinoa Salad with Mixed Greens, vibrant and refreshing on your palate. Each recipe was not just a meal but an adventure, an opportunity to explore and to grow. Consider, too, the challenges you faced. The days when time was a luxury you couldn't afford, when the call of convenience food was a siren song too hard to resist. Yet, here you are, having navigated those waters with the compass of your commitment guiding you. You learned that preparation is key, that a little planning goes a long way, and that the DASH diet, with its flexibility and focus on balance, fits into your life more seamlessly than you imagined. Now, look at your victories, both big and small. The morning you woke up feeling more energized, the compliments from loved ones noticing a change not just in your appearance but in your aura. The scales that tell a story of pounds lost, sure, but more importantly, of health gained, of blood pressure numbers that slowly edged into the realm of 'normal', whispering promises of a future filled with possibility. As you stand here, at this juncture, it's crucial to look forward, to peer into the horizon of your continued journey. The road doesn't end here; in many ways, it's just beginning. You've laid the foundation, now it's time to build upon it, to expand your culinary repertoire, to explore new flavors and textures, to continue learning about the nutrients that nourish your body and soul. The next steps are yours to decide. Maybe it's committing to trying one new recipe each week, exploring the local farmer's market for seasonal produce, or perhaps it's a deeper dive into understanding the nutritional science that underpins the DASH diet. Whatever path you choose, know that it's paved with the knowledge you've acquired and the experiences you've gathered along the way. But beyond the food, beyond the recipes and the meal plans, this journey is about you. It's about setting an example for your family, showing them that a heart-healthy lifestyle is not just possible but enjoyable. It's about the conversations around the dinner table, where you share not just meals but stories, laughter, and love. It's about community, about sharing your journey with others, inspiring them just as you've been inspired. Embrace this lifestyle with the understanding that it's not about perfection but progress. There will be days when you stray from the path, when life's unpredictability makes adherence to the DASH diet challenging. Forgive yourself for these moments, for they are not failures but part of the human experience. Use them as stepping stones, learn from them, and continue forward with renewed vigor. As you move into this next chapter of your journey, remember that change is a constant companion. Your needs, preferences, and circumstances will evolve, and so too should your approach to the DASH diet. Stay open, stay curious, and most importantly, stay committed to your health, for it is the greatest gift you can give yourself and those you love.

13.2 How to Adapt the DASH Diet as a Long-Term Lifestyle

Imagine for a moment the stories of those who have walked this path before you. There's the tale of a busy mother of three, juggling work, family, and her own health. Initially, the DASH diet was a lighthouse guiding her through the fog of dietary confusion. Over time, it became her north star, a constant in the chaos of daily life. Through trial and error, she learned to weave the principles of DASH into the fabric of her family's meals, finding that balance between health and happiness, between the rigidity of rules and the fluidity of life. Then there's the story of a man in his mid-sixties, facing the reality of hypertension and the risk of heart disease. For him, the DASH diet was not just a recommendation from his doctor but a lifeline thrown in turbulent waters. As he navigated this new way of eating, he discovered a passion for cooking he never knew he had. The kitchen became his laboratory, where whole grains, lean proteins, and a rainbow of fruits and vegetables were ingredients for both his meals and his rejuvenation. These stories, while unique, share a common thread—a deep understanding that the DASH diet is more than a list of foods to eat and avoid. It's a journey of discovery, of learning to listen to your body, to honor its needs while delighting in the pleasures of nourishing food. This understanding is the key to transforming the DASH diet from a temporary eating plan into a sustainable way of life.

Adapting the DASH diet for the long haul involves embracing flexibility. Life is unpredictable. There will be celebrations and sorrows, busy days and lazy weekends. The secret to sustainability is learning to bend without breaking, to make choices that align with the spirit of DASH even when strict adherence is impossible. It means enjoying a slice of birthday cake without guilt, then returning to your usual eating habits with the next meal. It's about finding joy in the journey, not just the destination. Sustainability also hinges on simplicity. In the rush of modern life, complexity is the enemy of consistency. Streamlining meal planning and preparation, relying on a core set of ingredients that can be mixed and matched in endless variations, ensures that healthy eating doesn't become a burdensome chore. Remember, the goal is to weave the DASH diet into the tapestry of your life, making it as natural and effortless as breathing. Community plays a pivotal role in this adaptation process. Just as a single thread is weak on its own but strong as part of a tapestry, so too is our journey strengthened by the support of others. Share your journey with family and friends, not just as a way of explaining your food choices but as an invitation for them to join you on this path. Find or create a community of fellow travelers, sharing recipes, tips, and encouragement. Together, you'll discover that the road is easier and far more enjoyable. Education is another cornerstone of making the DASH diet a lifelong companion. The principles of healthy eating are constant, but our understanding of nutrition evolves. Stay curious, stay informed, and be willing to adjust your sails as new information becomes available. This doesn't mean chasing every dietary trend but rather deepening your understanding of the principles that underpin the DASH diet, allowing you to make informed choices that align with your health goals and lifestyle. Finally, integrating the DASH diet into your life for the long term is about celebration. Celebrate the flavors of fresh, wholesome food, the energy and vitality that come from nourishing your body, and the small victories along the way. Celebrate the moments of connection over shared meals, the traditions you'll create and pass down, and the legacy of health you're building for yourself and those you love.

13.3 RESOURCES AND SUPPORT FOR CONTINUING YOUR DASH DIET JOURNEY

Embarking on the DASH diet journey is akin to setting sail on a voyage towards improved health and well-being. As you chart this course, it's crucial to have a compass and a map — resources and support that will guide you through the ebbs and flows of dietary change and help maintain your new lifestyle. Imagine you're on a journey, not just any journey, but one that promises a treasure trove of health benefits. The DASH diet, your chosen path, is more than a diet; it's a lifestyle that nurtures your heart and body. But like any explorer, you need a toolkit to sustain this venture.

This toolkit comprises resources and support networks that act as your North Star, guiding you towards continued success. First, let's talk about the kind of support that makes a difference. Community plays a pivotal role in our lives, and it's no different when adopting a new eating habit. Engaging with local and online DASH diet communities can offer you a sense of belonging. Picture yourself sharing recipes, success stories, and challenges with others who are on the same path. These interactions not only motivate but also enlighten, as you discover the myriad ways people integrate the DASH diet into their diverse lifestyles. Moreover, healthcare professionals, such as dietitians and nutritionists, are invaluable allies. They're like the seasoned guides who know the terrain by heart. Consulting with them can provide personalized advice that aligns with your health needs and goals. They can help you navigate the complexities of meal planning, ensuring that your diet remains balanced and enjoyable. Now, let's delve into the treasure trove of resources available at your fingertips. Books and cookbooks specifically about the DASH diet are your maps, detailing the routes to take for a heart-healthy lifestyle. They offer a wealth of knowledge, from scientific research behind the diet to a plethora of recipes that cater to various tastes and preferences. Imagine your kitchen shelf stocked with these books, each one a gateway to a new culinary adventure that doesn't compromise on flavor or health. In the digital age, the internet is a treasure chest waiting to be unlocked. Websites dedicated to the DASH diet, blogs penned by nutrition experts, and online forums buzzing with discussions provide a wellspring of information. Through these platforms, you can access the latest research, find answers to your dietary questions, and connect with a global community of DASH diet enthusiasts. Cooking shows and online video tutorials bring the DASH diet to life in your kitchen. Watching chefs prepare DASH-friendly meals can be both educational and entertaining. These visual guides demystify cooking techniques, making healthy eating seem less of a chore and more of a creative endeavor. Technology also offers a bounty of tools to assist in your journey. Mobile apps that track your dietary intake, provide recipe suggestions, and monitor your progress can be your digital companions, helping you stay committed to your goals. They serve as your personal diary, charting your journey and celebrating your milestones along the way. Remember, the journey on the DASH diet is not just about following a set of nutritional guidelines; it's about creating a sustainable, enjoyable lifestyle. Therefore, it's important to find resources that resonate with you personally. Whether it's a cookbook that speaks to your culinary style, a community that welcomes you, or a mobile app that fits seamlessly into your daily routine, the right resources can make all the difference in your journey.

www.ingramcontent.com/pod-product-compliance
Lightning Source LLC
Chambersburg PA
CBHW081553250726
48653CB00009B/3407